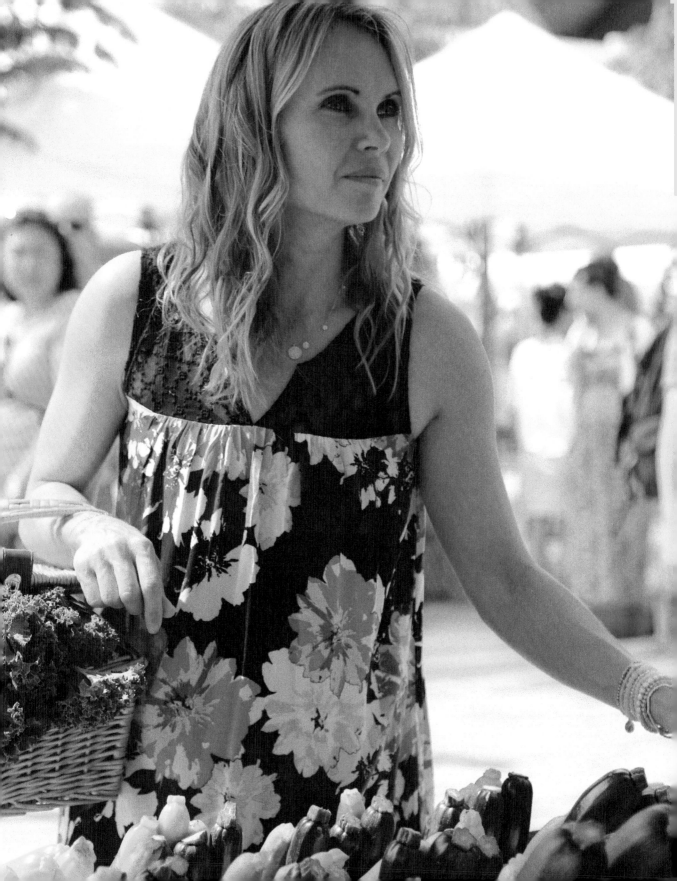

FOREWORD

There are nutrition experts who value the importance of nutrition and food and there are nutrition experts who create delicious recipes to do that. Rarely do you see the two in one passionate individual. But so it is with Michelle Vodrazka.

Both on and off the stage Michelle educates, inspires and teaches others on both solid nutrition values AND applies those principles in easy, delicious recipes. An incredible expert, mother of four and peer, I am so happy and honoured to recommend this book to anyone searching to eat a little healthier, happier and NOT count a single calorie.

May I personally suggest the Raw Strawberry Mini Cheesecakes? Trust me. You will thank me later. Thank you Michelle for continuing to embody health and happiness to me and all you come into contact with.

Kathy Smart

North America's Gluten-Free Expert
Best Selling Author, TV Show Host
Owner of Live The Smart Way Expos across Canada

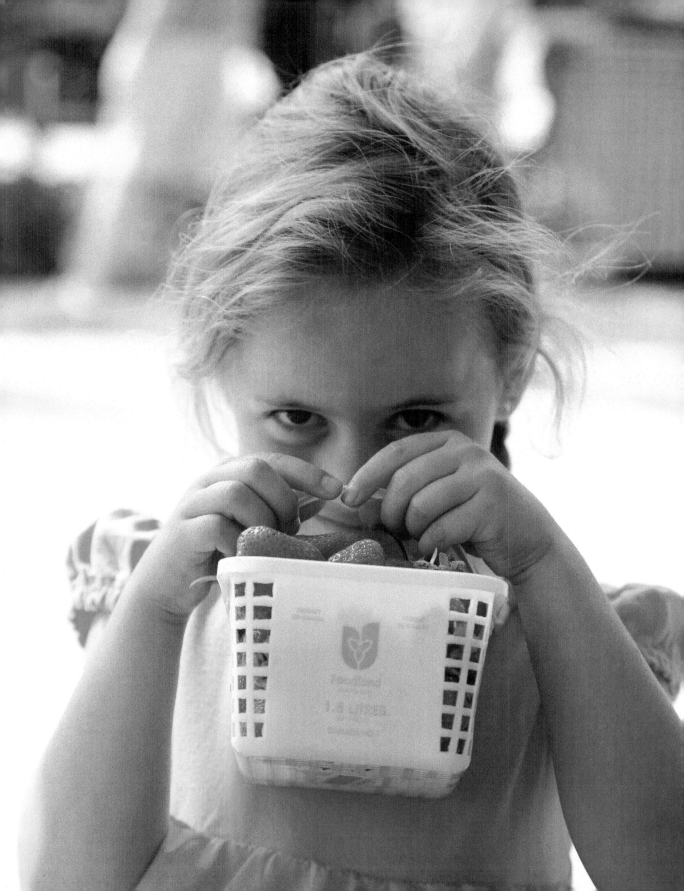

INTRODUCTION

Welcome! I am so excited that you have chosen to embark on this trip into wellness with me. My own path into wellness is constantly evolving as I continue to learn from my mentors, my fellow health warriors, and my amazing clients. I am always humbled by the incredible support that exists in the health-and-wellness community and how willing people are to help each other succeed and thrive, and I feel incredibly lucky to have been accepted into this amazing community.

Now to you, my fellow readers, who are the main reason why I wrote this book. You have inspired me to create recipes that not only taste good, but that will make you feel good and look good, too. Every single human being deserves to know how it feels to be healthy, confident, and full of energy. My mission is to help you discover new ways to cook, eat, and move, so that you can reach your full potential and live the life that you have always dreamed of living. I know that it can be scary and overwhelming when you are first starting out, but here's the deal — you don't have to be perfect! Nor do you have to get it right every time.

In fact, I encourage you to get it wrong sometimes. Perfection is over-rated — and boring. Sometimes the best discoveries are born out of our mistakes. Mistakes are how we learn best and they help us grow. I can't tell you how many recipes in this book were created out of mistakes — and somehow, they always turned out to be the best-tasting ones! In fact, I thought I had my entire philosophy about health figured out when I was 19, then I thought I re-figured it out at 28, then again at 38, and guess what? At 40 years of age, I still don't have it figured out. One thing I do know is that you can overdo anything, even things that are healthy, and when we get too caught up in dictating that there is one perfect way to be, or act, or live, or eat, then we miss out on some of the most magical moments in life.

Now, there may be times, like the time in my life that you will read about in the next chapter, when it's necessary or desirable to hone in on your health (or the health of a loved one) with a laser-like focus — even at the expense of falling out of balance in other areas of your life. These points in life, such as when faced with a health crisis or when training for a competitive event, might require an incredibly high level of commitment. You may need to let go of other things that bring balance (and perhaps also joy) into your life for a short period of time, which is okay. Just remember that when you leave other areas unattended for too long, they may wither, and your health may end up being adversely affected.

So as regularly as you can, take care of your body and feed yourself well, but also remember to take care of your mind and your spirit. When we take care of others all the time, we use up our own energy, and if we don't refill our "buckets", we end up getting burned out, ill, or depressed. So take the time, ideally each day, to refill your bucket. Sometimes that simply means doing what feels most pleasurable in that particular moment. Sometimes it means taking the time to relax and breathe, or to do things that bring you pure unadulterated joy.

Let go of the idea of the perfect life, the perfect house, the perfect presentation, the perfect diet, or the perfect workout program, because there is no such thing. Focus more on the moment, on what is right in front of you. Enjoy the beauty of a simple sunset, a warm bath, a steaming cup of coffee, a good sweat, an incredible goal, a cuddle with your pet, a kiss from your child, a joyous laugh, a bright bowl of berries, a slow walk in the woods, a perfectly ripe avocado, or a gorgeous heap of greens picked fresh from your garden.

What this book is meant to do is give you some tips and tricks and, of course, to provide you with some amazing recipes that will make it easier for you to be healthier without feeling like you have to make great sacrifices to get there. When you eat, move, and live in a way that brings you pleasure and simultaneously supports your health, then, my friends, you have the recipe for an amazing life. As Brian Wansink says in his book *Mindless Eating*, "the best diet is one that you don't know you're on."[1] So read on to learn how to make healthy living as fun and joyful as possible.

My Journey into Wellness

My journey into smoothie-loving, green-juice-drinking, kombucha-making, kale-and-quinoa-eating, glass-water-bottle-using, and from-scratch-cooking was like waking up to find yourself in a foreign country where no one speaks your language. Even though sometimes I wish it had been more of a natural evolution over a length of time, I am glad that it happened this way, because it compelled me to re-evaluate the way my family was living.

I still remember the exact day my world changed forever. It was February 18, 2011. I had been experiencing numerous health issues for years before, symptoms that plagued me, but that did not reach the medical threshold for concern, so no doctor could give me any answers to my increasingly strange and depressing health problems.

I suffered from numerous stomach issues (constant pain, gas, bloating, and frequent bowel movements), joint aches, and fatigue so severe that I could barely manage to get out of bed in the mornings. I knew I needed help, but I couldn't find anyone who could help me, so I just started to resign myself to the fact that I would feel this way forever. I wish I could say that I had some great awakening, but the day that I changed my entire life had nothing to do with me. It had to do with my then barely one-year-old daughter, Noelle. I blogged about the day my world changed several years ago, and the details are still so raw that I prefer to repost what I wrote back in 2013 than have to rehash them over again, so here it is:

> *This post has taken me two years to write. It is by far the most difficult and the most emotional post I have ever written. I still remember the exact moment that my blood went cold and I realized there was something very, very wrong with my youngest daughter, Noelle. The realization chilled me to the bone. All of a sudden, it became clear that we were losing her — losing the smart, funny, sassy, little baby girl who had charmed us from the moment she graced us with her first smile and delicious giggles.*
>
> *Up until she was 12 months old, she had been developing along a path similar to that of my other three children, hitting her major milestones, smiling, laughing, crawling, and talking, and then taking her first steps. She was an incredibly cuddly baby, who loved snuggling up to me, crawling all over me, and putting on a show for attention from her brother and sisters.*

Then, shortly after her first birthday and her 12-month vaccinations, the connection we had with Noelle started to disappear. She smiled less, her laughter became infrequent, her eye contact diminished and she slowly lost her newly acquired words — "Mama", "Dada", "ball." We became helpless bystanders as we watched the light in her eyes disappear.

Then it got worse. She refused to be touched anymore and would cry if we tried to pick her up or cuddle with her. She started playing by herself in a corner, opening and closing kitchen cabinets over and over again. She even started dragging her right leg behind her as she walked, and she began to constantly lose her balance. Then her left arm started hanging at her side almost uselessly, with her elbow constantly bent, and her increasingly deteriorating fine-motor skills became a huge source of frustration for her and an endless source of heartbreak for us. By February 18, 2011 we felt as if we had completely lost her.

We were presented with a slew of possibilities, from Rett Syndrome (a truly horrible disease) to autism. Although it would take us several more months to get a diagnosis, I knew in my gut that it was autism that had robbed her from us. In the same way, I also knew she was still inside the fog that had started to encase her and I knew that I had to find a way to get her back. I knew that I could not stop — that I would not stop — until I had dragged her back out of the fog, and helped her find her way back to this world and back to her family.

So what did I do? I opened my computer and started googling everything to do with autism. I googled autism research, autism cures, autism conferences, autism treatments, diets for kids with autism. I spent days reading, researching, and creating lists of resources in Ottawa. Then I started calling doctors, psychologists, specialists, schools, and hospitals, and placed my daughter on waiting lists. There were waiting lists for everything — waiting lists to talk to specialists, waiting lists for schools specializing in autism treatments, waiting lists for psychologists, and waiting list for doctors.

The result of all of this intense effort was very discouraging. Many of the waiting lists for autism treatment covered by our health care system were two or even three years long, and costs for private assessments and treatment centres were exorbitant. For the first time in my life, I didn't care what these services cost and I was ready to take out a second mortgage to pay for the treatments that I felt would give Noelle the best tools and the best chance to make it back to our world. Even so, we had to wait several months for Noelle to be assessed privately.

In the meantime, I was supposed to be patient and wait, but my gut told me that if I sat idly by while we waited, she would just drift further and further away from us. So for the next 12 months, I made it my full-time job to harass people (nicely of course) to ensure that no one would be able to forget that Noelle was on their waiting lists and cancellation lists. I also immediately changed her diet.

With the help of a local doctor who treated kids with autism, we removed gluten, dairy, yeast, and sugar, and we started feeding her foods that could help heal her gut. We also started her on a pretty aggressive supplement regime, trying to provide her with as many nutrients as we possibly could to help her body (and mind) heal itself. We had her on numerous vitamins,

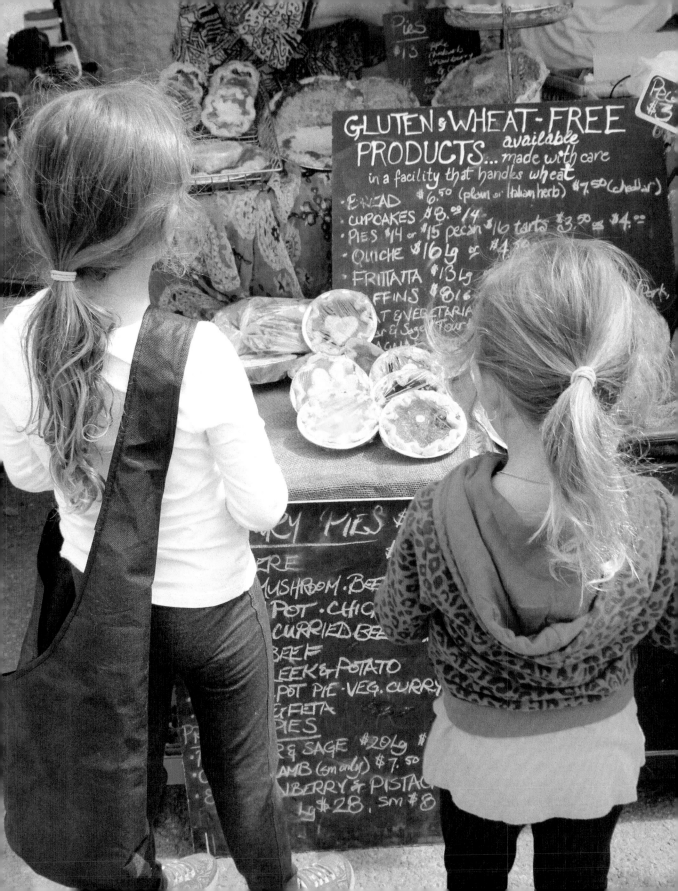

minerals, probiotics, fish oils, and digestive enzymes, just to name a few.

In the meantime, we got in to see the doctors. Noelle received a provisional diagnosis of PDD NOS, which is a form of autism. We were told that she would never live independently, that she would likely never talk again, and that our outlook was bleak. We briefly thought of placing her in a full-time school for kids with severe autism, but I was so disheartened by what I saw when we visited that I just couldn't do it.

Although science seemed to show that behavior therapy was one of the top interventions for children with autism, it just didn't feel right to me. All I could think was that if we put her in one of those schools, she would never come back to us, and we would lose her for good. She needed to be in a regular school, with a variety of children from all backgrounds, not just children who had severe autism. I felt that this was the best chance to get her back, while her mind was still so pliable.

So while we waited to be accepted into the program of speech therapy, occupational therapy, and social work at the Ottawa Children's Treatment Centre (OCTC), I did more research. If I had chosen to believe the science, I would not have bothered to change her diet. The scientific studies all show that there is minimal to no improvement for children with autism by diet change alone, but since we had nothing else to do but wait until we were able to access any treatments, I felt that we had nothing to lose. Plus, there was a ton of anecdotal evidence that a change in diet did help, and it gave me hope, which I held onto like my life depended on it (because my daughter's life did).

So we threw out everything in our cupboards — literally everything — and we started from zero. I knew that to compel dramatic changes in Noelle's mind and body, we needed to make dramatic changes in our diet and our way of living and that we needed to do it as a family. We already had been eating what I thought was a pretty healthy diet, but when I look back now, I cringe. We thought fat-free meant healthy, that canola oil and corn oil were good oils to use, and that it was healthier to drink 'diet' beverages because they had no calories.

Luckily, my husband was on board, because within ten days of changing only her diet and making no other changes, we started to notice a flicker of light in Noelle's eyes, a fraction of a moment here or there where we were able to catch Noelle's attention again. It was so fleeting that at first I thought I was imagining it, grasping onto something where nothing existed. These moments were so short that by the time we could point them out to each other, she had already disappeared and withdrawn back into her own world again — but we had what we needed: we had hope.

From there, our journey took 18 more months until we welcomed Noelle back into our world. With the help of an amazing daycare who provided Noelle with extra help, OCTC, a tiny bit of speech therapy, an amazing doctor who adjusted Noelle's supplements as required, and a new diet, we battled our way back. Noelle's motor skills improved and she stopped falling over, her leg stopped dragging behind her, her arm relaxed again at her side, she started making eye contact with us again, and her smile returned. Her words slowly came back and she started talking and interacting with her siblings again.

It was a long, hard journey, but Noelle was finally back in our world again. Finally we could breathe again, and work on the small issues that remained from having missed out on almost two years' worth of normal childhood development. Now I am sure there are many people out there who will claim that Noelle was misdiagnosed from the start, and that is fine with me. We know what we saw, we know what we experienced, and we have our daughter back — and that is all that matters. Only my family and I can know the fight that we have battled, the long and treacherous journey we have endured, and the changes that have unfolded under our eyes. We still have the battle scars to prove it, but it was all worth it because in the end, we emerged victorious.

Now, I want to make it clear that I am not saying that what we did will work for anyone else or in any other situation. It is up to you to determine what feels right to you, and what you are willing to do. I have found that people often think they are willing to move mountains if they or their loved ones were to get sick, but in reality, not everyone is able to put in the huge amount of time and massive effort that is required to create an environment which will allow the body and the mind to heal, nor is everyone interested in, or open to, challenging conventional medical wisdom. Plus, I believe that we had a few additional things working in our favour.

First, we were lucky that we had three other kids, because we were able to notice something was wrong really early on in Noelle's development. With autism, the earlier you intervene, the better the outcome. Second, we were able to be incredibly strict with her diet. You see, after talking to several other families who said that a diet change did not work for them, I found out that some were still relying on processed foods, and their diet changes were often short-lived because of the massive learning curve and intense effort that this type of overhaul required. Third, we had the financial resources to be able to pay for all of her supplements and for nutrient-dense, organic foods.

It's important to remember that children (or adults for that matter) who are fighting their way back from disease need to ensure that every single morsel of food that enters their mouth is as nutrient-dense as possible. Simply going gluten-free and dairy-free is not enough. Now, I am sure that there are other families who have done everything that we did, and more, and still didn't have the outcome that we had. All I can say is that each of us is unique and all of our bodies and minds respond to different stimuli, in different ways, and at different rates. So be patient, never give up hope and never stop researching and trying new approaches.

You may be surprised to learn that I thank my lucky stars each day that this happened to us, because it compelled me to start feeding my family better and to appreciate each and every moment on this earth. Noelle's battle inspired me to learn about nutrition and cooking and it served to remind me to be more present in my life. It even helped encourage me to start taking ownership for my own health and to learn how to heal my own body, a little bit at a time. The way I see it, Noelle actually saved my life and for that, I am forever thankful.

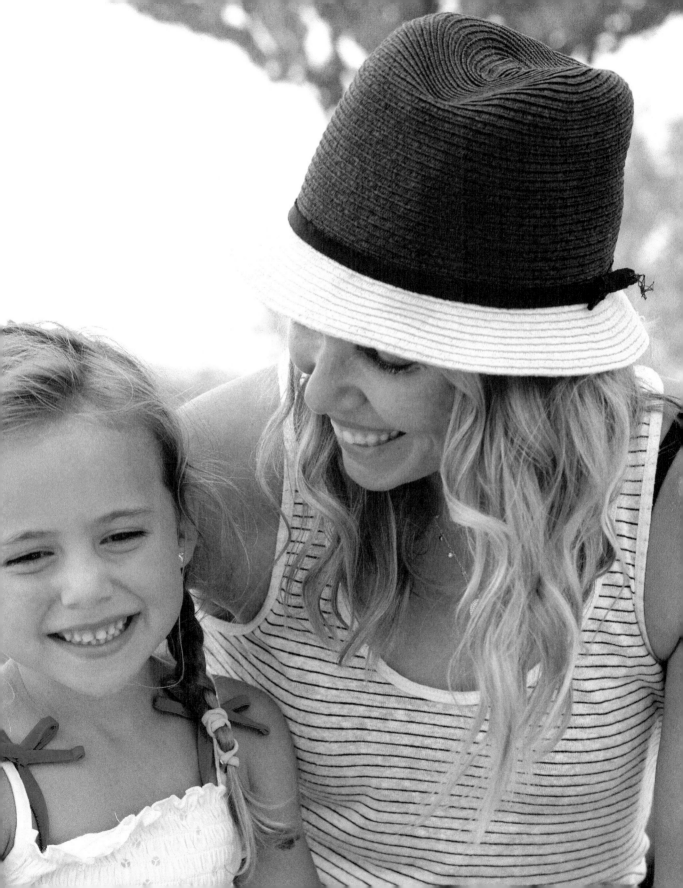

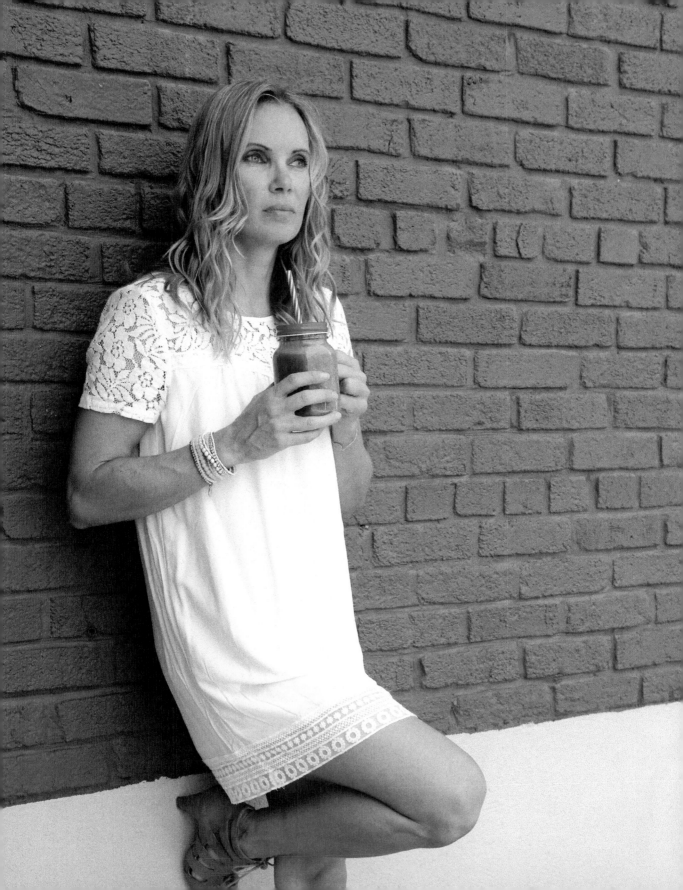

WHY HELP YOURSELF TO SECONDS?

The concept behind *Help Yourself to Seconds* was based on the fact that for 90% of people, calories don't matter, and so you can help yourself to seconds — if you eat the right things. You may initially scoff at this idea, but I have tested this theory with hundreds of clients. If you eat the right things, at the right times, then how much you eat ceases to matter, because your body will self-regulate itself and get what it needs to help you look and feel your best, which includes maintaining a healthy bodyweight.

Now, what we need to do is define what a healthy bodyweight is. A healthy bodyweight is a weight that provides you with relentless energy, booming self-confidence and maximum protection against illness and disease. It is not about the last ten "vanity" pounds and it is not about having a six-pack. If you want to achieve those things, then you probably *will* need to measure out portion sizes, and you will need to be a bit more militant about what you are putting into your mouth. But who wants to live like that long term? Certainly not me, although I have to admit that in the past, I have competed in numerous fitness competitions sporting an impressive six-pack.

The point is, I ate that way for a short period of time to achieve a certain look, but it certainly wasn't fun, nor easy, nor did it help me support optimal health. There is just no possible way to obtain all the nutrients your body needs when you are in a caloric deficit or on a very low-calorie diet. That is why fitness competitors have "on seasons" and "off seasons", and why competitors need to allow time for their bodies to recover after competing.

Now back to the way the rest of us folks live our lives. Most of us want to eat in a way that supports our health and allows us to feel our best. We want to eat in a way that allows us to have lots of energy and to be able to perform well in our chosen activities. We want to eat in a way that doesn't require too much effort, and yet allows us to maintain a healthy weight. We want to feed our children in a way that allows them to thrive and in a way that provides them with the nutrients they need to grow and to learn. We also want to eat in a way that gives us pleasure and joy, where the food we prepare tastes delicious and looks beautiful.

The recipes in this book allow you to do that. I have taken care to create each and every meal so that it is as nutrient-dense as possible without compromising on taste. In fact, the recipes in this book are so delicious that you will have a hard time believing that they are actually good for you. When we eat the right things, and focus on the most nutrient-dense foods in the world, they fill us up and satisfy us because they are naturally low in calories and high in fibre. In contrast, when we eat junk foods (calorically dense, nutrient-void foods), our bodies will keep craving more food until we get the nutrients we need. You see, our bodies are pretty smart that way.

The right foods also provide our bodies with nutrients that act as enzyme inductors (they either speed up enzymes, slow them down, or induce the manufacture of more enzymes). These enzymes affect all the hormonal and metabolic processes in the body. When we have the right enzymes, operating at the right speeds, our metabolism is optimized, our hormones are balanced, and we are able to burn fat and build muscle more efficiently. Furthermore, eating the right things at the right times is always going to be more important than how many calories we eat. The old adage that *calories in equals calories out* is a thing of the past.

One of my dreams is that we would all live in a world where fresh, local food was readily available, where there was little food packaging and processing, and where we all enjoyed preparing and cooking our own food. If that were the case, we would not need to worry about figuring out what the claims on food labels actually mean, and we wouldn't have to wonder what so many unintelligible ingredients were doing in our food. What is scary is that while food production is increasing (it's now a 1.6 trillion-dollar-per-year industry[2]), the nutritional value of our food keeps decreasing. We now have packages with mile-long ingredient lists and minimal nutritional value.

The result of this is that we are over-fed and under-nourished. In layman's terms, this means that even though we are fatter than ever, our bodies are still starving. In fact, most of our grocery store shelves are filled with food-like products that don't contribute to our health but that instead contribute to disease. To make matters worse, sugar is now being added to 80% of the processed food on US grocery store shelves[3] (and I bet Canada is not much better). We have gotten so used to all of this excess sugar that we have lost touch with what food tastes like in it's natural form, and thus lost our desire for real, whole, unprocessed food. In fact, Michael Moss, author of *Sugar, Salt, Fat: How the Food Giants Hooked Us*, claims that the high-sugar, energy-dense, fatty, salty, junk food that can be found on our grocery store shelves are specifically tailored to keep us addicted to these foods through neuro-chemical addiction[4].

Now, before you start to feel helpless and betrayed by the big, bad food industry, remember that you have a choice and a voice! You have the power to vote with your dollar and stay away from these artificial food-like products that have no place in our bodies anyway. If we return to the basics, and simply take a few moments to reflect on where food our comes from, then it becomes harder to justify buying or eating food products that don't even resemble anything close to the natural state of their ingredients. If you look at some of the foods in your household, can you discern where it was grown or how it got there? If it needed to be transformed and processed in a plant, as opposed to having been grown naturally on a plant, how can it be used for building and healing your body?

Unfortunately the power of food has been long forgotten. We need to remember that food should be respected, acknowledged with gratitude, and prepared with love. One hundred and fifty years ago, all of our food was organic and local and mainly prepared within the home. One hundred and fifty years ago, cancer and heart disease were also incredibly rare. Now, cancer and heart disease affect one out of three people and one out of two people, respectively. We have to ask ourselves why. Why do we insist on feeding ourselves food or food-like products that we know are bad for us? When are we going to take responsibility for the harm we are causing ourselves? A recent study showed that through diet and exercise alone, we could cut breast cancer by 50%[5]. Now, that's way better than any other treatment option that exists today, yet most of us would rather pop a pill than eat more vegetables.

Another study showed that the average middle-age weight gain of 22 pounds increases our risk of a heart attack by 75% and increases our risk of breast cancer by 50%[6]. Yet another study showed that female cancer survivors could cut their mortality rate from 16% to 4% in a 10 year period, just by engaging in moderate exercise such as walking two miles most days a week and eating five fruits and vegetables a day[7]. What you eat and how you move have a far greater impact than you may think.

We have 100 trillion cells in our bodies[8] that are made out of what we eat. We are replicating ourselves based on information in the food that we are eating, and yet we wonder what went wrong and why we got sick. Yes, there are other factors involved, like lack of movement and fresh air, increased exposure to toxins and pollution, and stress (among others), but the way we feed ourselves is a major part of the problem and one we can control. Every bite you take has the potential to either fight disease or feed disease, so choose wisely.

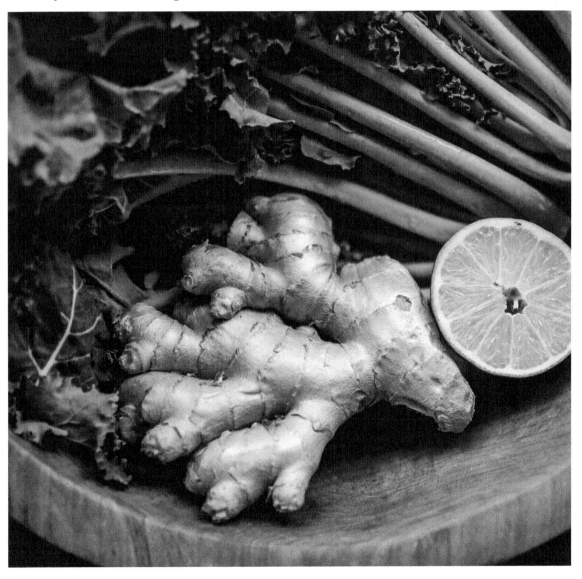

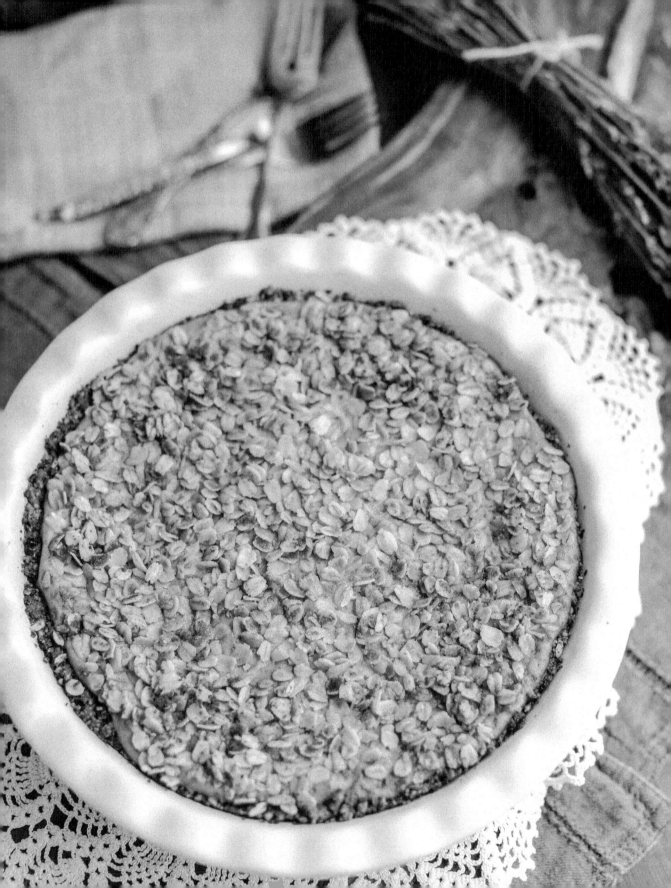

NUTRITIOUS, DELICIOUS WELLNESS

Why We Eat What We Eat: The Food-Mood Connection

Now let's get to the real reason why we (in North America) eat the way we eat. My mentor Cynthia Pasquella, who is the best transformational nutrition coach I have ever worked with, has a saying that really captures our emotional connection to food. Although it's true that you are what you eat (and digest and absorb), it's also true, as Cynthia says, that "*You eat what you are.*[9]"

What she means is that the way you eat is a reflection of how you feel about yourself. This also helps to explain why we sabotage ourselves and why we continue to make the choices that we do, even though we know what we *should* be doing. Feeling unworthy and unlovable and using negative self-talk will lead us to make negative food (and life) choices, because we don't think that we deserve to have good things happen to us.

Thinking that "*If only I could lose weight, then I would...*" is setting yourself up for failure. Although you may initially achieve the weight loss, if you don't learn to love yourself as you are *now*, and learn how to be happy *now*, then your self-worth and happiness will always be reliant on external factors. The truth is, self-worth and happiness come from inside of you, from your perspective and your outlook on life, and if you don't learn to be happy now and love yourself as you are now, then you certainly won't love yourself when you lose weight, get that amazing job, or meet an incredible guy....Get my drift?

Instead of piling on the self-love (which is what we should be doing), we judge ourselves and use negative self-talk; we say things like "*I am disgusting,*" "*I am so fat,*" "*Why am I such a failure?*" or "*No one could ever love me.*" Casting such harsh self-judgment and making unkind comments is incredibly counter-productive because they are a self-fulfilling prophecy and can serve as an excuse for not achieving your goals. If you find that you continually talk to yourself this way, then it becomes easy to never follow through on losing the weight or making the changes you want to make. "*Why bother?*" becomes a really easy fallback.

You see, most of the time, this feeling of inadequacy, this negative self-talk stems from our past, and a lot of time it starts in our childhood. We are told that we are "*too this*" or "*too that*" or that we need to "*stop being like this*" or "*stop doing that*" — ""*You are too emotional,*" or "*Stop being so loud.*" Essentially, we are told that WHO we are is not good enough and that the WAY we are is the WRONG way to be. We hear it from our parents, our teachers, our classmates, and later, our bosses, our partners, and even our own selves. So we are left believing that we need to act a certain way or look a certain way in order to be accepted and loved. We are led to believe that we are not good enough just the way we are.

Instead of judging yourself or allowing others' opinions to dictate your self-worth, try to accept yourself as you are. Accept that you are on an evolutionary path, a path of growth, and that you won't be perfect, but that you can start choosing a different way to be, choosing a different way of responding to your stimuli. Instead of re-acting (or acting unconsciously), try to start making conscious and mindful choices. Sure, you may stumble and fall back into your old patterns, but instead of judging yourself (that was bad/good, right/wrong, I failed/succeeded), accept that you are not perfect and ask yourself why you behaved that way or why you made that choice.

So what if you ate a bag of chips and a pint of ice cream? So what if you prepared poorly and gave a terrible presentation? So what if you ran a terrible race? Does that make you a bad person? No! We terrorize ourselves and cast such harsh judgement on ourselves. Think about it: How would you act if this happened to your friend? You would probably empathize with them and be extra supportive, and you would likely gently help them to move on. So why do we judge ourselves in such a harsh manner? In these circumstances, try to treat yourself like you would treat your best friend. Be compassionate, be kind, and be understanding. Give yourself some leeway, because you are human after all, and therefore, as my teacher Cynthia Pasquella likes to say, "You are perfectly imperfect.[10]"

Rest and Digest vs. Fight or Flight

Being kind to yourself also extends into the way you live the rest of your life. If you are always putting yourself last, running yourself ragged, and taking on too much without taking time to recover, you will eventually hit a wall. Ignoring your basic human needs, whether it's for love and physical affection, relaxation and recuperation, passion and purpose, joy and happiness, or health and well-being, will catch up to you. It might start to manifest itself in the form of physical symptoms, such as an illness, fatigue, weight gain, or pain, in the form of emotional symptoms, such as crying spells, withdrawal, or emotional volatility, or as psychological symptoms, such as anxiety or depression. If you continue on this way, these symptoms will eventually become louder and more serious, until you have no choice but to listen.

The key is to take the time to notice these signs before it's too late and to take action, instead of sweeping them under the rug and pretending they don't exist. We can work hard and be successful, but we also need to balance it out by making time to laugh, love, play, and rest. We have created this crazy culture where being busy has become a status symbol which we wear as a badge of honor because we equate it with success. But here's a little secret: being busy does not mean you are successful, and being successful does not mean you are happy or healthy.

We have also become a culture of constantly needing more — more power, more money, more stuff, more distractions, and more activities, and for what? We are sicker and more stressed than ever. We need to redefine what success means to us as a society (Arianna Huffington has written extensively about this in her new section in the *Huffington Post* called the *Third Metric: Redefining Success Beyond Money & Power*). Do we really need all this stuff to be happy? I venture that we don't. So why are we killing ourselves to get more of it?

So what are the repercussions of always being busy? Well, living a life where you are constantly on-the-go, where you have a never-ending to-do list, and where you have minimal time for yourself, means that you are operating in a mode known as the *Fight or Flight* mode. This mode is switched on as an automatic reaction to stress and danger and is managed by the sympathetic nervous system. The sympathetic nervous system is the part of the nervous system that is responsible for controlling involuntary bodily functions, such as your breathing, your heart rate, and your digestion. This response was originally designed to ensure our survival as a species. It would turn on in a critical, dangerous situation, such as when a very hungry saber-tooth tiger appeared from behind the bushes while we were out gathering berries. When faced with this type of threat, our body would get ready to either fight or to flee, by preparing itself to act fast, minimize damage and preserve (our) life.

Luckily, or unluckily, depending on how you look at it, we've inherited these responses from our prehistoric ancestors. When faced with a stressful situation, our adrenal glands immediately produce the stress hormones epinephrine (adrenaline), norepinephrine (noradrenaline), cortisol and aldosterone, our heart rate and blood pressure increase, our breathing gets faster, our pupils dilate, our awareness intensifies, our perception of pain diminishes, our blood sugar levels increase, and our blood is shuttled away from the skin, the digestive system, and the reproductive organs in order to increase blood flow to the heart and the working muscles. In this mode, we see everything as a potential threat to our survival.

Now these are all fantastic protective mechanisms which come in real handy when we're about to get mugged, when we're faced with a bear, or when we need to pull one of our kids out of the path of a speeding car. The problem is that our nervous system can't distinguish between a real or an imagined threat, and it doesn't know if that threat is due to an angry-looking bear, or a bad day at work, a fight with a loved one, money problems, horrendous traffic, negative self-talk, or the stress of being constantly busy, so our body reacts the same way to all of these threats. Now the key is not to completely get rid of all the stress in our lives. In fact, a little bit of stress can be beneficial because it helps us get out of bed in the mornings and helps motivate us to get things done.

However, if we maintain that feeling of stress for days, weeks, or even months, apart from the immediate effects on our physical state (difficult digestion, lowered libido and reproductive hormones, decreased fat-burning, elevated cortisol levels, and high blood sugar) we're also making our organs work overtime to keep up with that (unnecessary) threat in the long-term. This is not the state that you want your body to be in for a prolonged period of time, as some of the diseases strongly linked to sustained stress include cancer, hypertension, cardiovascular disease, autoimmune disease, diabetes, ulcers, PMS, hypertension, anxiety, and depression.

The mode that we should be spending most of the time in is a state of *Rest and Digest*. The *Rest and Digest* response is managed by a subdivision of the autonomic nervous system called the parasympathetic nervous system. This division is also known as the D division, which is defined by its most important roles: digestion, defecation, diuresis (urination). We activate this response when we feel safe and when we are joyful, happy, relaxed, calm, and at peace. In this state, our bodies can relax. Our heart rate and blood pressure return to normal, our hormones fall back into balance, and our body can focus on digestion, reproduction, fat loss, healing, and yes, even pooping.

Now, this is where I want to be 95% of the time. What about you? If only it were that easy, right? In this modern world, we barely have time to catch our breath, much less restore and relax. We are so busy *doing* that we forget what it means to just *be*. We are so busy accomplishing things that we forget to pause and enjoy what we have achieved. The question is, how do we activate the *Rest and Digest* mode if we don't have conscious control over it? Well, we can create an environment where our *Rest and Digest* mode gets activated. Here are some tips to get you started:

- When you are eating, try to do just that: eat. No distractions! No TV watching or internet surfing, no working, no studying, no driving, and no standing. Take a seat and focus on enjoying your food and chewing it thoroughly.

- Practice deep breathing or do some meditation, which is one of the best ways to activate the body's relaxation response and help move you into the *Rest and Digest* mode.

- Do some mild, gentle, low impact, mind-body exercise, like yoga or tai chi, which can stimulate our feel-good hormones and make us feel happy and relaxed.

- Spend some time outdoors and in the sunshine. We are connected to nature at the cellular level and it makes our minds and bodies feel calm and happy.

- Do more things that bring you joy, like dancing to music, playing with the kids, taking a bath, reading, or laughing, and do less of the things that cause you stress or make you unhappy.

- Try journaling and writing down the things you are grateful for. Feeling grateful makes us happier, and when we are happy, we stimulate our parasympathetic nervous system.

- Avoid processed foods, foods that are high in sugar, and foods you might be sensitive or intolerant to (these foods cause internal stress in your body).

- Get enough sleep. Going to bed by 10 pm[11] and getting at least 7–8 hours of sleep a night can help us combat the effects of stress[12].

- Be realistic and don't take on more than you can handle. Learn that it's okay to say no, and to do so without any explanation whatsoever. My good friend and meditation teacher, Luc Blanchard, taught me this one.

- Outsource what you can and ask for help. Building a good social support network is key in maintaining optimal health and decreasing stress. Remember, it takes a village!

- Give back to the community. Giving back to others is good for decreasing stress levels because it increases oxytocin, which is a feel-good hormone that helps the body relax.

Incorporating some of these tips into your life will help bring the *Fight or Flight* and the *Rest and Digest* modes into better balance. Remember, the key is to make sure you are not being overly dominated by your *Fight or Flight* mode, which is unfortunately the mode that we have gotten used to spending a lot of time in. One really important aspect of staying in *Rest and Digest* mode for our long-term health is eating mindfully, which we will jump into next.

Eating Mindfully:
It's not just what you eat, it's how you eat

So what does it mean to eat mindfully? Eating mindfully means being fully present and eating with *intention* and *attention*. Eating used to be a natural, healthy, and pleasant experience that was shared with our families and our communities, but that's a far cry from the fast-paced, distracted, on-the-go way we eat our meals today. Have you ever experienced looking down at your plate only to realize that you have already finished what was on it and yet you are left with no recollection of how it tasted? Talk about a pleasure killer!

Furthermore, distracted and rushed eating can lead to numerous digestive problems such as indigestion, gas, cramping, bloating, diarrhea, constipation, and over-eating, among others. The good news is that eating mindfully is really quite simple to do and the benefits are substantial. Eating mindfully can improve digestion, reduce over-eating, increase our enjoyment of food, lead to a better relationship with our food, and stimulate weight loss. So next time you sit down to eat, try to incorporate some of these tips:

1.   Keep a food-mood-hunger journal. You can download a copy of the journal that I use with my clients on my website at www.michellevodrazka.com/food-mood-journal. Knowing whether you are eating because you are hungry, tired, sad, or upset, can be a really useful tool to help you change mindless eating patterns.

2.   Skip the convenience foods and learn how to prepare your own food in your own kitchen. There is nothing quite like the hands-on experience of making your own food to help you connect to the sights, smells and feel of your food. It also helps us connect to where our food came from.

3.   Avoid over-eating by eating off of smaller plates. The larger the container (or plate) that the food is served in, the more we tend to eat (about 18% more in fact). So switch out your dinner plate for a salad plate and if you are thinking about refilling your plate after you have cleared it, pause to consider whether your body really needs to eat more.

4.   Learn how to plate your food so that it is visually appealing. A plate that looks beautiful and is full of colors gives us a greater appreciation for what we are about to eat. The more appealing our food looks, the more likely we are to savour it.

5.   Sit down at your table to eat and turn off all distractions. Instead of eating standing up, at your desk, in your car or in front of the TV, sit down at your dining room table and tune in to your food. You get bonus points if you can sit down at the same time as the rest of your family or your living companions.

6.   Have an attitude of gratitude. Before you eat, take a moment to think about where your food came from, the energy that went into harvesting it, the love that went into preparing it, and the gratitude you feel for getting to enjoy it.

7.   Tune in and pay attention by using all of your senses. Notice what your food looks like

and smell its aroma. Feel the texture of your food as you put it on your mouth, and notice the multitude of flavours and sensations as you chew, and savour each and every bite.

8.   Slow down between mouthfuls and chew your food properly. Take time to pause between bites (maybe even set down your fork) so that you can notice when you are satisfied and avoid eating to the point of fullness.

Kicking Cravings

Now that you are being more mindful, maybe those cravings that you have are becoming more noticeable. I bet that just by the mere mention of cravings, you can picture, even smell, the food that you regularly crave. Let me guess, for most of you it's something sweet, perhaps chocolaty. For others, it's something salty and fatty like chips or cheese. Did I nail it? The foods we crave are normally high in calories, carbohydrates, and fat, are usually consumed in large quantities, and have little protein content. We also usually only have about two or three trigger foods, foods that seem to have more control over us than we have over them.

Know that you are not alone: it is estimated that 70% of men and nearly 100% of women suffer from food cravings[13]. The top four triggers of food cravings that I see in my practice are nutrient deficiencies, fatigue, emotional triggers, and blood-sugar imbalances, so let's take a closer look at each of these in more detail.

Due to the poor quality of our soil there has been a decline in the amounts of vitamins and minerals in our fruits and vegetables over the past half century. In fact, in a study published in the *Journal of the American College of Nutrition*, researchers found that between 1950 and 1999 there had been reliable declines in the protein, calcium, phosphorus, iron, riboflavin, and vitamin C content of 43 different types of fruits and vegetables.

Combine this decline with the long transit time that it takes for our food to travel from farm to fork (an average of 1500 miles), and we have even greater nutrient depletion. Plus, with the highly-processed Standard North American Diet (SAD) that we are eat today, most of us are not even coming close to eating the recommended eight to ten servings of fruits and vegetables each day. When your body lacks nutrients, it will crave more food to try to meet its macro and micronutrient needs.

Fatigue is another common reason for food cravings, particularly for foods that are high in stimulants like sugar, caffeine, and refined carbohydrates because they give us a jolt of energy. Unfortunately these "uppers" are always followed by a "downer" when our body crashes. What most of us fail to understand is that what our body really needs is rest and sleep and not an artificial stimulant. Research shows that in order to prevent cravings and keep our hunger hormones in balance, we need a minimum of seven hours of sleep a night, and up to ten or even twelve hours if you are an athlete[14].

Emotional triggers are another reason why we eat the way we eat, but sometimes we aren't aware of the connection because eating to stuff down our feelings has become such an ingrained, automatic habit. When we feel bad, we crave foods that are fatty and sweet because we know that they will make us feel good by acting on dopamine receptors (our feel good chemicals) in the brain. To break the emotional eating cycle, start by paying attention to what you are feeling when a craving strikes or use the food-mood journal mentioned above.

I saved the big one for last. Blood-sugar imbalance is one of the most common triggers for food cravings and can lead to a vicious cycle of bouts of high energy followed by a crash of no energy. All sweets and starches get converted into glucose, which causes our pancreas to release insulin to remove the sugar from our blood (the high) and draw it into our cells. The resulting drop in blood sugar due to the insulin release makes us tired again (the low), so we crave sugar and simple carbs because our bodies have learned that they provide us with quick energy.

Take time to pay attention and see if you can figure out which of the above triggers are responsible for your cravings. That way, you will build the awareness to start changing these ingrained patterns and, hopefully, begin responding differently.

Trade Up Instead of Giving Up

Having worked with hundreds of clients over the past five years, I have learned a thing or two about change psychology. One of the most critical lessons I have learned when it comes to helping people change their eating habits, or any habit, really, is that the moment you tell someone that they can't eat (or do) something, all they want to do and all they can think about is the very thing you told them *not* to do. See, once we perceive that our free will and our ability to choose is being restricted, we automatically rebel.

No one likes to be told what to do. We didn't like it as children, and we certainly don't like it as adults, so why do we continue to go on diets where we are told that we cannot eat this or have that? Even when we set these restrictions ourselves, our minds still rebel against them. Oh, I can't have any more Reese's Peanut Butter Cups? Well, we'll see about that! And out we go to the store to buy a pack of Reese's Peanut Butter Cups (or we send our partner out for them). It's the same thing that happens when we go on a severely calorie-restricted diet. Our bodies and our minds get scared that we will be entering a time of scarcity and so our body enters into starvation mode and starts shutting down all but the most necessary systems.

On the other hand, the other side of the spectrum is not much better. When we have too much choice and too much abundance, we become gluttons. So the answer seems to lie somewhere in the middle. Allow freedom of choice, but don't lay out a buffet every night. Instead of restricting all bad foods, provide healthy alternatives that don't make people feel deprived. The secret is to focus on the good stuff that you want more of, because eventually, the good stuff will slowly and effortlessly start to crowd out the bad stuff.

Obviously the recipes in this cookbook are a great place to start, and I've worked hard to upgrade a lot of your favourite dishes, but I know you won't always be cooking from scratch. So, in addition to the awesome recipes in the second half of this book, I have provided you with a handy table that will help you see how easy it is to trade up your favourite not-so-healthy supermarket foods for more nutritious versions.

Instead of this . . .	Choose this . . .
Bottled water	Fresh spring water, mineral water, infused water or filtered water from home
Breakfast cereal or store-bought granola	Homemade granola, whole grain porridge, or oatmeal with nuts /seeds
Candy	Medjool dates, frozen grapes, figs, or ginger chews
Canned beans	BPA-free canned beans or dried beans
Canned creamy soup	Puréed soup or homemade soup with some coconut milk
Canola, corn, soy, cottonseed or sunflower oil	Coconut oil, avocado oil, extra-virgin olive oil, grass-fed butter, or ghee
Chocolate chips	Dairy-free chocolate chips or carb chips
Coffee	Herbal, caffeine-free coffee alternatives, or green tea
Coffee creamer	Vanilla almond milk, coconut milk, or coconut cream
Commercial jam	Chia-seed jam or double-the-fruit jam
Conventional milk	Nut or seed milks, sheep's milk, goat's milk, or if you tolerate dairy, organic cow's milk
Conventional store-bought dips	Homemade hummus, pesto, or salsa, or natural nut butters
Fries	Baked potato, sweet potato or turnip fries
Frozen or take-out pizza	Whole-grain fajitas with pesto sauce and pizza toppings or cauliflower crust pizza topped with pesto and veggies
Frozen yogurt	Banana "nice" cream, smoothies, smoothie bowls or homemade frozen yogurt made with coconut milk
Fruit yogurt	Unsweetened coconut yogurt, sheep's milk yogurt, goat's milk yogurt, coconut kefir, or, if you tolerate cow's milk, unsweetened organic plain yogurt, Greek yogurt, or kefir
Gatorade	Homemade sports drinks, coconut water, diluted fruit juice with a pinch of sea salt, or green tea with honey
Ice cream	Coconut ice cream or banana "nice" cream
Iceberg lettuce	Kale, baby spinach, romaine lettuce, Boston leaf lettuce, watercress, cabbage, or spring mix
Juice	Fruit and herb-infused waters, mineral water, freshly-squeezed fruit and veggie juices, or herbal teas
Ketchup	Hot sauce or salsa
Margarine	Grass-fed butter, ghee, or coconut oil
Mayonnaise	Homemade mayonnaise, hummus, mashed avocado, Dijon mustard, pesto, or Greek yogurt if dairy-tolerant
Microwave popcorn	Homemade stove-top popcorn made with coconut oil or ghee, and sea salt
Milk chocolate	Dark chocolate (70% or more cacao)

Instead of this . . .	Choose this . . .
Nutella	Store-bought chocolate-hazelnut butter or homemade chocolate spread
Popsicles	Frozen bananas dipped in chocolate, frozen homemade smoothies, or frozen grapes
Potato chips or popcorn	Store-bought seaweed chips, kale chips, sweet potato chips, or homemade popcorn drizzled with coconut oil
Processed parmesan	Nutritional yeast or freshly-grated, aged, hard parmesan, if you are dairy-tolerant
Pudding cups	Avocado pudding or chia seed pudding
Regular peanut butter	Natural, unsweetened almond, peanut, coconut, hazelnut, or cashew butter
Sandwich bread	Portobello mushrooms, romaine lettuce, or collard greens
Soda pop	Mineral water, fruit-infused water, or kombucha
Store-bought cookies	Homemade cookies, healthy mug muffins, or baked oatmeal
Store-bought muffins	Homemade muffins; a piece of fruit with a handful of nuts, or nut butter
Store-bought salad dressing	Freshly-squeezed lemon juice, apple-cider vinegar, or balsamic vinegar with olive, avocado, or flax-seed oil, or homemade dressings and vinaigrettes
Store-bought sauces and marinades	Hot sauce, tamari sauce, liquid aminos, lemon juice, lime juice, herbs, or spices
Store-bought snack bars	Homemade energy bars, fresh fruit with nut butter, dried figs, dried dates, or homemade trail mix
Store-bought bouillon	Organic broth or homemade stock
Store-bought trail mix or dried fruit	Trail mix made without refined oil, unsulfured dried fruit without any added sugar, or roasted chickpeas
Whey protein powder	Vegan protein powders like pumpkin, brown rice, or hemp powders, or grass-fed whey protein powder
White bread	Minimally processed gluten-free, whole-grain breads, collard-green or romaine lettuce wraps, or portobello caps
White flour	Brown rice, buckwheat, quinoa, coconut, almond, arrowroot, or oat flour
White pasta	Quinoa, buckwheat or brown rice pasta, zucchini noodles, shirataki noodles, or spaghetti squash
White potatoes	Sweet potatoes, butternut or buttercup squash, cauliflower, carrots, or turnips
White rice	Brown, black, or wild rice, millet, or quinoa
White sugar	Coconut palm sugar, sucanat, pure maple syrup, raw honey, applesauce, bananas, date paste, or prunes

Foods That Don't Deserve to be in Your Body

Although I believe that you can eat almost anything you want in moderation, there are certain foods that really have no place in your body. Regular and sometimes even moderate consumption of the following foods has been linked to obesity, depression, early aging, lack of energy, high blood pressure, nutrient deficiency, heart disease, cancer, and diabetes.

Please understand that in general, I don't think it's smart to apply "good" and "bad" labels to foods; however, the following foods really do cause more harm than good, and I don't think you can technically even call them 'food". In fact, "food-like product pretending to be a food that is intended for human consumption" might be more accurate, so I have no problem placing them on a naughty list. These are foods your body would not miss if you never ate them again.

Please note that there are many, many treats that I have not added to this list. For example, *homemade* cakes and cookies are not on my naughty list because they do not contain ingredients that cause damage to your body if eaten in *moderation*. I believe that as long as they don't contain harmful ingredients, like those listed below, occasional treats have their proper place in a diet otherwise filled with fresh, nutrient-dense foods. Treats can provide us with sensory satisfaction and pleasure, both of which are important aspects of leading a well-balanced life.

So, without further ado, here are the top five foods that don't deserve to be in your body:

1. **Non-fat foods:** Usually contain artificial sweeteners (the worst!) or added flour, sugar, and salt. Instead, try 2% or full-fat versions of these products; a little fat is good for you and it will taste way, way better.

2. **Processed and packaged cakes, cookies, and crackers:** Contain added sugar, salt, chemicals, preservatives, and trans-fats. Instead, bake your own or at least buy them fresh from a local bakery.

3. **Processed meats:** Contain nitrates and preservatives and can harbor dangerous bacteria. Plus, they were recently labeled as carcinogens by the World Health Organization. Instead, try fresh meats, canned or fresh fish, beans, and natural nut butters.

4. **Soft drinks:** Contain sugar, high-fructose corn syrup (or sweetener), sulphites, artificial food colors, and tons of calories (unless you opt for the "diet" version, but then you get artificial sweeteners to contend with). Instead, drink regular or sparkling mineral water or herbal tea.

5. **Artificial sweeteners:** These are the worst! Have I said it enough times yet? And, I feel your pain, because did I mention that I used to be totally addicted? Yup, me. I had the worst diet-cola/sugar-free gum habit in the free world. Never again. You neither!

6. **Crappy supplements**: This is a bonus one for you. There are so many poor-quality supplements on the market these days that contain all kinds of questionable ingredients.

Do your due diligence by reading the labels and researching the company. Check for any artificial sweeteners, flavours, colours, and fillers and see if there were any recalls, customer complaints, or lawsuits filed against the company. High quality supplement companies usually invest in independent, third-party testing, and they often have links to research backing their supplement claims on their website.

Putting the Puzzle Together

Changing your diet can seem like a huge endeavor. So what should you do whenever you are faced with something that seems so large and so overwhelming that it practically paralyzes you? You break the task down into teeny tiny pieces (like a puzzle) and you start to put those pieces together one by one. To build a solid nutritional plan, there are several pieces you can start with, right away, that will change the way you look, feel, and even behave. It's up to you to decide which piece you want to start with. Just keep in mind that the easiest and fastest way to start noticing a difference is simply to *take action* by implementing just one thing.

"Sounds great", you say, "let's do this!" ...But instead of diving in and choosing something big, like most of us tend to do, I'd like you to pick something *easy* and *small* that you can commit to doing *every day* for the next *two weeks*. If there is any doubt in your mind that you will not be able to do it, then pick something else you know you *can* do. For example, your puzzle piece might be to eat one serving of vegetables at every meal. If you feel very confident (as in you are 90% sure) that you can do this every day for the next two weeks or until it becomes a habit, then that's where you start. However, if you are not sure you can commit (say you are only 75% sure) then you need to go back and pick an easier starting point .

What you do not want to do is to overhaul your entire way of eating and living and make the change so overwhelming that you just give up. Remember that willpower is finite and it will run out when it's overtaxed, so focus on making just one small change at a time. Starving yourself and eating less than a thousand calories a day may give you results fast, but in the long run, it will also lead to malnourishment, binging, a sluggish metabolism, a loss of existing muscle mass, and a host of other health-related issues, not to mention a huge likelihood that you will abandon your plan in a few weeks (most people have this all-or-nothing approach to eating, which is just a blueprint for failure).

What you need to remember is that all the pieces that you are putting together are part of a bigger picture. These small pieces will eventually build on top of one another seamlessly, so that when you turn around a few months from now, you will realize that you have created a whole new lifestyle. Think about it! If you were to change just one habit every two weeks, by the end of the year you would have developed 26 brand new habits! That's a completely different life, my dears. Now, if that's not a puzzle worth putting together, I don't know what is.

So now I'm sure that you're racking your brain, wondering where to start and which puzzle piece to choose first, so I have provided some examples below. This is nowhere near an exhaustive list; it is only meant to provide you with some inspiration. The piece that you pick needs to be an individual choice based on your current condition, goals, and lifestyle.

PLEASE REMEMBER:

Choose only one change at a time;

Ensure that it fits with your goals;

Make sure it is action-based and not outcome-based;

Pick something easy (almost too easy);

Choose something you can do daily;

Set up your environment for success;

Don't delay, start doing it right now;

Track your progress each day;

Keep it up for two weeks;

Be patient and don't expect perfection;

Once you nail it down, repeat all steps;

Remember adding one new habit every two weeks equals 26 new habits a year;

Check out your brand new life!

SOME PUZZLE PIECE IDEAS:

Start your day with a healthy smoothie.

Eat three servings of vegetables a day.

Try a new healthy recipe every day.

Eat a serving of protein at every meal.

Record what you eat in a food diary.

Eat a large salad for lunch.

Go to bed at 10 pm each night.

Be active for 30 minutes a day.

Eat sitting down without distractions.

Eat only until you are 80% full.

Make your dinners from scratch.

Drink 6–8 glasses of water a day.

Walk for 15 minutes each day.

Bring your lunch to work.

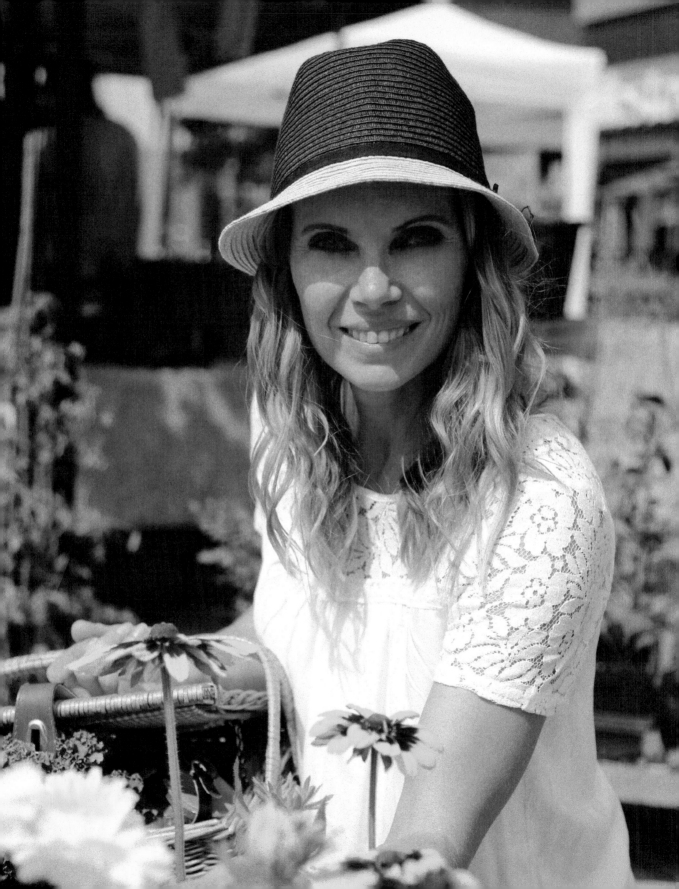

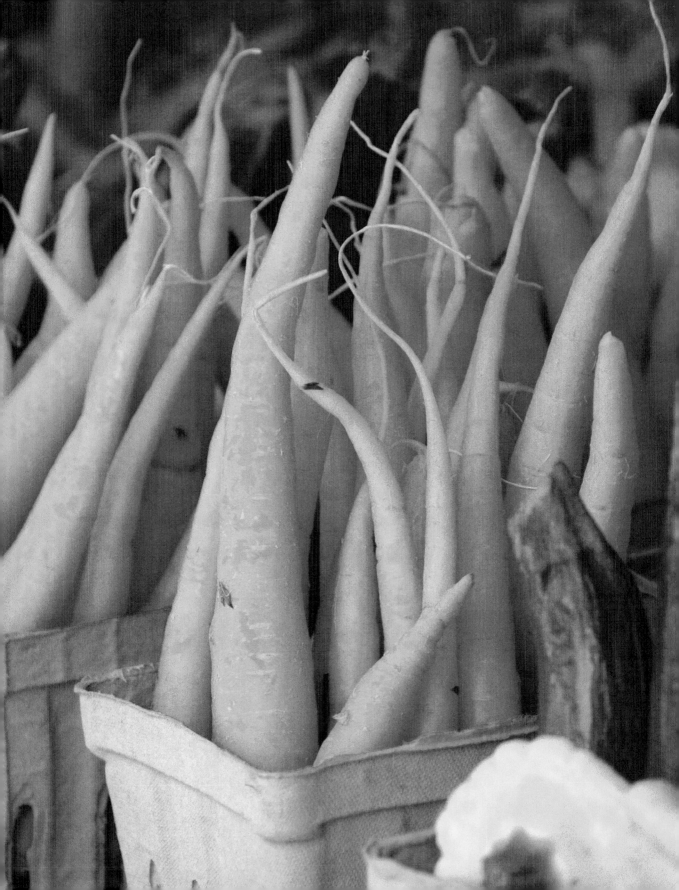

CHANGE IS HARD...
LET'S MAKE IT EASIER

I want to start off by saying that if you are not truly ready to change, then it won't matter how much knowledge you have, or how great your nutrition plan is, or even how small and easy your new habit is, because you won't end up sticking to it. Being ready for change requires commitment, consistency, preparation, flexibility and the willingness to accept responsibility for your behavior. Even if you are someone who enjoys and embraces change, the initial adjustment period is always going to be difficult because so much is unknown.

Humans are creatures of habit and when we don't know what lies ahead, we get anxious, nervous and scared. These feelings are normal, so acknowledge them and maybe even write down what you fear the most. Are you scared of failure or success? Are you nervous that your relationships might change? Are you experiencing discomfort due to lack of control? Are you worried about what people will think? Being aware of your fears and anxieties will help you to move past these feelings in a productive manner and enable you to focus on actually making the change.

Once you are ready to make a change, the best piece of advice I can give is to repeat what I already said: take baby steps. Ease your way into your new lifestyle slowly. Research shows that when people try to make even just two changes at once, they are only 35% likely to be successful[15]. However, if you stick to one change at a time, your odds of success shoot up to 85%[15]. So start focusing on one small, easy habit, and commit to that habit 100%.

Remember, success builds success; that's why it's important to start small. Once you have incorporated a single habit into your life for two or three weeks, you can incorporate another one. Don't try to do it all at once because chances are, you will fail. Even when I start to diet down for a competition, I don't jump into a new style of eating all at once; I ease my way into it. Each month, my diet slowly gets stricter and my body and mind are able to ease into the challenge gradually (and prepare for what comes next), because it is happening at an acceptable, almost indiscernible pace. This way, I stay physically healthy and mentally sane.

The second crucial piece of advice regarding adhering to your new plan is to shape your environment for success. Making a lifestyle change is hard enough, so don't make it harder on yourself by testing your willpower at every turn. Remember, willpower (the act of self-control) is finite. This is one of the reasons that most people tend to blow their diets in the evening. You may not even be aware that you are depleting your willpower throughout the day – resisting the candy bowl at work, not yelling at your kids when they don't listen for the 100th time, standing up to your boss, finding motivation to make it to the gym – all of these things use up your willpower so that at the end of the day it becomes very, very hard to resist temptation.

My advice is, don't try. Set up your environment in a way that makes it easy to succeed. Don't keep treats or junk food in the house. Go to bed half an hour early so you don't snack in front of the TV. Lay out your workouts clothes before you go to bed. Set up a basement gym so that working out is convenient for you. Keep your fridge stocked with healthy meals. Enlist support from your family and friends beforehand so that they don't sabotage your efforts. Help yourself succeed by setting up your environment for success.

The third piece of advice is to take the time to learn your weaknesses and make them work to your advantage. For example, if your limitation is that you lack social support, do something about it. Engage your partner and get them excited about your new lifestyle. Maybe recruit them to be your workout partner or challenge them to a fat loss contest. If it's your friends that are sabotaging your efforts, make some new friends that lead healthy lifestyles and plan get-togethers around activities rather than meals. Online communities (like facebook groups) and social media feeds can be another incredible source of support, motivation and education.

If you have a hard time fitting your workouts in, then break your workouts into mini fitness sessions throughout the day, or schedule them into your calendar along with all of your other appointments. If you are having a hard time getting motivated, join a sports team or hire a coach to write your nutrition and training plan for you. As you can see, there are many ways to work around your limitations, but you need to be aware of them so that you can build a sound mitigation strategy to deal with them.

Finally, if all else fails, don't underestimate the power of distraction. Humans are not as good at multi-tasking as most people think they are. Since the human brain prefers to process only one thing at a time, distraction is a powerful tool you can use to divert your attention away from something unhealthy (like junk food, a craving, or a bad habit) towards something more positive. Physically relocating to a new environment (like taking a walk or having a nap) or mentally engaging in a new task (like knitting, reading, or calling a friend) can stop cravings and bad habits in their tracks.

Kick Your Metabolism Into High Gear

I have been telling you all along that if you eat the right foods at the right times, calories don't matter and that you can help yourself to seconds. Now, that is true 90% of the time. However, there is a time when calories may come into play, and that is when you are in the domain of vanity pounds — when your diet already consists of high-quality foods, when your weight is already in the healthy range, and when your goals are centered primarily on how you look. During these times, it may be wise to watch your portion sizes and to stick to a single serving, but even in this case, what you eat and when you eat still trump how much you eat. If you want to learn more about nutrient timing, I speak about it in the Q & A section of my first cookbook, *Smart Snacking for Sports*.

Fat loss is actually quite simple. [Insert loud snort here]. "Right," you're thinking, "if fat loss is so easy, why am I having such a hard time losing fat, and furthermore, why are there are so many books, programs, and supplements on the market today, each claiming to have the 'real' secret to weight loss?"

The answer is that there are many, many reasons why people have a hard time losing fat, and figuring out what your personal limitations are (your social support system, your environment, your motivation, etc.) is a really important step towards being successful in achieving your fat-loss goals (I need to write another book to get into all this). Although losing fat is not hard, sorting through all of the information on the market today, and figuring out what is based on real science and what is based on fiction, can be dizzying.

The reason that the weight-loss industry is a huge multi-million dollar market is that people take advantage of the fact that losing fat *seems* difficult and complicated and people can become very rich from promoting their products and supplements. The bottom line is, many of these products and diets *do* work — in the short term — because most of them require a reduction in your total caloric intake while generally recommending an increase in activity levels. However, there is often no lasting fat loss because many of these programs are either unrealistic, unsustainable, expensive, too restrictive, too fast-paced or just totally bogus.

So before you follow any of these programs, spend a lot of money, and possibly negatively affect your long term health, let me share my secret (for long-term fat loss) — for free! My secret is, that there is no secret. Fat loss is not complicated. We humans are complicated and our lives are complicated. But we never used to need help from anyone — we didn't need the government, or dietitians, or nutritionists, or personal trainers, or books, or the internet — to tell us how to eat. We just instinctively knew how to feed our bodies.

So what happened? Life got complicated — and busy. Food got complicated, and fast, and profitable, and fake. Now it seems like you need a PhD to know how to feed yourself properly. It's crazy. So, let me just give you some simple tips that will help you get back to the basics, so that you can become a lean, mean, fuel-burning machine, all without ever having to count a single calorie.

Caveat: If you want to get your body fat down into the single digits (think six packs and fitness competitors), you may need more specific guidance than what I am going to provide you with in this book. However, for a healthy, lean, fit-looking body, just follow the tips below. Now I'm not saying it is going to be easy, but if you can stick to the guidelines below 90% of the time, you'll get 90% of the results. Now that's pretty good in my book (get it, "in my book"?).

Tip #1: Eat every 2–3 hours or, don't. Let me explain. Eating every few hours is not going to increase your metabolism (as many people claim), but by eating smaller meals more frequently, you stabilize blood sugar and energy levels and you minimize hunger. This means you are much less likely to have cravings, and your desire to reach for foods that are high in calories and low in nutrition (literally "junk foods") will diminish. Furthermore, because your meals will be smaller, your body will have an easier time absorbing most of the calories and putting them to good use supporting your body's processes as opposed to storing them as fat for future use.

However, if you are one of those people who has a hard time not snacking, then it might actually benefit you to stick to three square meals a day. I have a lot of clients who are grazers whom I have taken off of snacks, and immediately they started shedding weight that they hadn't been able to lose for years. Only you know what works best for you.

Tip #2: Include vegetables, fat, and lean protein in every meal. Vegetables provide you with the nutrients you need to keep your metabolic processes functioning properly and the fibre you need to keep you full longer (and help you detox properly). Protein is necessary for building muscle, muscle tissue is more metabolically active than fat, and fat will provide your meal with flavour and satiate you in a way that other macronutrients can't.

Tip #3: Save your carbohydrate-heavy meals for after you exercise. Following weight training or High Intensity Interval Training (like sprinting, plyometrics, tabata, etc.), there is a short period of time when your insulin sensitivity is heightened and your body's ability for tolerating carbs increases. This means that those carbs will be put to good use building muscle tissue and are less likely to be stored as fat. If your goal is fat loss (as opposed to muscle building or maintenance) it's ideal to stick to complex carbs (such as quinoa, sweet potatoes, brown or wild rice, whole grains, oatmeal, etc.) during this post-workout period. If you are going to eat carbohydrates at any other time during the day, make sure they are in the form of fruits and vegetables, with a strong emphasis on vegetables. An ideal post-workout meal would include a balance of carbs and protein at a ratio of 3:1.

Tip #4: Include a good balance of healthy fat in your diet. This means a balance of saturated, monounsaturated, and polyunsaturated fats. You are already likely getting the saturated fat if you include meat and dairy in your diet, so you likely only need to focus on meeting your unsaturated fat requirements, which can be found in fatty fish (like wild salmon, sardines, mackerel, herring or anchovies), olive oil, nuts, seeds, and avocados, to name a few. Healthy unsaturated fats will also help to keep you motivated, boost your mood, and elevate your metabolism. A good ratio of omega-3 to omega-6 fats is 1:1[16]. Unfortunately, in this day and age of highly processed convenience foods, most of us are getting a ratio of 16:1 or 20:1[16] — not good! I recommend including healthy fats at each meal, especially omega-3s —except during your post-workout meal, where you want to focus primarily on proteins and carbs. A great explanation of omega-3 and omega-6 fats can be found at www.precisionnutrition.com/all-about-fats[17].

Tip #5: Be aware of your portion sizes. This is especially essential if you are trying to get lean, which is important, because leaner people live longer (see, it's not just about the looks). A serving of protein for women is about the size of your palm and about two palms for men. A serving of fat for women is the size of your thumb and about two thumbs for men. A serving of complex carbohydrates for women is about the size of a fist and two fists for men. A serving of vegetables is anywhere from a ½ cup to 2 cups, although it is really hard to eat too many vegetables, so just keep them coming. You can download a copy of these visual portion size guidelines from the Precision Nutrition website at www.precisionnutrition.com[18].

Tip #6: Stay well hydrated. Stick to water, green tea, or herbal tea. It is also okay to have a daily coffee, especially pre-workout (depending on the type of caffeine metabolizer you are – see www.michellevodrazka.com/is-coffee-harmful-or-helpful-it-depends-on-your-genes), because it can provide you with an extra kick of energy. Beware, however, of letting the daily cup of java become one, then two, then three...until you become one of the people who needs their coffee to get going. Can you say "addict"? Furthermore, caffeine is a diuretic and dehydration can mimic hunger, so sometimes when we think we need to eat, it's really just that our cells are crying for some water! Metabolism and performance both drop when you are even mildly (2%) dehydrated because dehydration causes fatigue and affects muscle contraction — both of which are related to performance[19]. Why would you care about performance? Well, if you can't work hard at the gym, you won't be able to put in the effort you need to get the proper anabolic (muscle-building) response. Remember, more muscle = faster metabolism + a tighter body.

Tip #7: Do a minimum of three short, simple, and intense weight-training workouts a week. So this one's not nutrition-related, but if you really want to increase that fat-burning response, you need to lift heavy, lift with intensity, and lift efficiently. Lifting heavy can mean lifting your bodyweight (that's heavy enough!) or simply lifting heavy for you. It doesn't mean you need to be lifting gigantic dumbbells (although I do) or know the ins and outs of a squat rack, but if you want to get lean, you need to build some metabolic muscle tissue.

In order to boost your metabolism, you will need to lift with intensity, which simply means it should feel hard — for you. No sitting on the bench chatting for five minutes in between sets! Instead, you should be able to hit the gym (or the playground or somewhere you can throw heavy things around) and knock out your exercises in less than 30 minutes. Finally, you need to lift efficiently, which means sticking with exercises that provide a lot of bang for your buck, like pull-ups, push-ups, squats, lunges, deadlifts and kettle-bell swings. The only caveat I will give here is if you struggle with adrenal fatigue or burn-out. In that case, activities that are gentler on the mind and body may be more appropriate here, such as yoga, Pilates, leisure walking, and so forth.

Tip #8: Be active daily. Start by making an effort to move more. It's the little things that really add up and make a big difference. Pretend that elevators don't exist, park further away from the building, and spend a few more minutes outdoors enjoying the sunshine and fresh air. Clean your house. Ride your bike to the store. Do yoga. Shovel snow. You get the point. Eventually, as you get more advanced, you can add in some sprinting a few days a week. I am a huge fan of sprinting for one reason — actually, make that two: it gives you huge results and it will let you outrun the zombies one day.

Tip #9: Get enough sleep. Make a conscious effort to get to bed 30 minutes early. I guarantee you'll be surprised by the difference this makes. Studies have shown that those who sleep fewer than six hours a night gain twice as much body fat over a six-year period than those who sleep seven to eight hours a night. Sleep changes your hormone balance (in a favourable way) and provides time for your muscles to recover. Furthermore, when your body is tired, it craves energy, and that energy requirement can be satisfied by either sleeping or eating. If you stay up late, your mind will convince you that you need food for energy (even though what you really need is sleep) and you will end up consuming a bunch of calories your body didn't really need. Ideally, hit the sack between 10 and 11 pm and wake up between 6 and 7 am.

Tip #10: Opt for fresh food. Make sure your protein, carbohydrate, and fat choices are in the form of fresh, whole foods (see my recommended grocery list), which you will ideally prepare and cook yourself, in your own kitchen. If you do eat something that was pre-made (at a counter, restaurant, or grocery store) make sure to read the label first (a lot of the labels out there nowadays are scary!) and ensure that it is a nutritious, healthy choice. If you don't recognize the ingredients on the label, don't eat it, look the ingredients up, or refer to my list of *Top Nine Worst Food Ingredients*.

I'm doing everything right but I still can't lose weight

First of all, I want to point out that even the most knowledgeable, motivated, and focused athletes, who get paid big bucks (or small bucks) to stay in tip-top shape, don't do everything right — and here's why: They're human, and I don't know any human who is capable of being perfect 100% of the time. Plus, who is to say what is "right"? Just because it has worked for one person, doesn't mean that it will work for you, and just because it worked for you last time, doesn't necessarily mean that it will work for you this time.

Now that being said, there are certain general guidelines (see above) that will work well for most people, most of the time, and that will get them 80% of the way to their goals, especially when we're talking about fat loss. The problem is that sometimes we have blinders on when it comes to personal habits that are sabotaging our progress. So, to help provide you with some insight as to why you may not be losing weight even when you feel that you doing everything right, I have compiled a list of reasons why your progress could be stalling.

REASON #1: Sneaking bites here and there – Tasting food while cooking or baking, stealing bites off your kids' plates, licking the peanut butter jar, grabbing a candy, or three, out of your co-worker's candy jar — all these little bites can add up by the end of the day. I know this for a fact, because every time I write a cookbook, I gain five to ten pounds, just from constantly tasting my creations. Keep your hands to yourself and stick to your planned meals (unless you're writing a cookbook, in which case, taste away).

REASON #2: Relying too much on protein shakes or meal-replacement shakes – Your body requires many more calories to break down, digest, and absorb whole, fresh foods. Meal-replacement shakes are already processed and, due to their lack of fibre and micronutrients, are absorbed much more quickly by the body. Furthermore, processed foods (and liquids) don't release satiety signals the same way that whole, fresh foods do, so you may never get that "full" feeling most people search for after eating.

REASON #3: Chewing sugarless gum or drinking diet soda – Artificial sweeteners are some of the worst weight-loss saboteurs! They not only cause water retention and bloating but they also have been linked to sugar cravings and an increase in hunger signals, which lead you to eat more. Plus, it's important to retrain our taste buds so they can learn to recognize the natural sweetness in real foods (like sweet potatoes and carrots) again, and if you keep over-stimulating them and exposing them to artificial levels of sweetness, they will never be able to re-adjust.

REASON #4: Using too many condiments, sauces, or dressings – Ketchup, mustard, sauces, mayo, salad dressings, and dips are calorie-dense, nutrient-poor, and can contain a ton of sugar. Learn to enjoy the flavour of the food itself, and use fresh herbs and spices to enhance the inherent taste of your food, rather than relying on condiments, sauces, or dressings. It may seem hard at first, but if you give your taste buds a few days to adjust, you will be able to re-train them and learn to appreciate what real food tastes like.

REASON #5: Eating well during the week, but over-indulging on weekends – This is a very common problem for most people. They want to enjoy time with friends and family, and many of these get-togethers revolve around food which is of poor quality. Unfortunately, a weekend of indulging can undo all the effort you put in during the week. Next time you socialize, propose a different activity that focuses on being active, or just bring your own food. Once your friends and family get used to it, no one will make any comments anymore.

REASON #6: Having treats too often – A treat should be just that: an event or item that is out of the ordinary and gives you great pleasure. A treat should feel special and be reserved for special occasions only. Treats are not meant to be eaten on a regular basis — definitely not every day! It's also important to remember that you are consciously choosing to eat healthier; no one is forcing this on you. Be proud of your choice.

REASON #7: Skipping meals – Going too long without eating and letting yourself get over-hungry is a recipe for disaster, especially when it happens due to a stressful, busy day. Once you let yourself get over-hungry, you tend to make poor food choices and when you do finally get your hands on some food, you eat it so fast that you end up consuming way too much.

REASON #8: Over-doing cardio – Spending hours upon hours doing low- to moderate-level cardiovascular exercise will only make you hungrier, increase your cortisol levels, and catabolize some of your hard earned muscle mass. Stick to shorter, more intense cardio work, like High Intensity Interval Training (HIIT), sprint work, interval training, etc. Two or three times a week is plenty. Spend the rest of the time building some muscle.

REASON #9: Not resistance training – I'll say it again - resistance training is one of the best ways to increase your metabolism, change the shape of your body, and help keep the fat off for life. I will not work with a client who is not willing to engage in any type of resistance training because it is critical to long-term weight loss and good quality of life. If you're hesitant to hit the gym or find the weight room intimidating, then I highly recommend you try out a TRX which is one of my favourite pieces of equipment of all time. The TRX is a suspension training system which costs less than $200, gives you a kick-ass workout, and can be used anywhere (see www.trxtraining.com)[20].

REASON #10: Not working out with enough intensity – Lifting five- to eight-pound weights or participating in Zumba a few times a week is not going to stimulate your metabolism or help you increase your lean muscle mass (unless you are a complete beginner or a senior, or are recovering from an illness or injury). You need to move fast enough and resistance train with enough intensity that you are breathing hard and sweating.

REASON #11: Eating healthy foods without paying attention to portion sizes – Eating healthy food is great and should comprise the bulk of your meals; however, if your main goal is fat loss, you may also need to pay attention to portion size. I had one client who couldn't lose weight even though she swore she was only eating the foods on the healthy grocery list I gave her. I asked her to keep a food diary and I found out that she was consuming $1/2$ cup of nut butter a day! Just remember, there can be too much of a good thing!

REASON #12: Not being prepared – Always, always have some healthy snacks at home, in your purse, in your car, in your cabinet at work. Prepare your meals and snacks ahead of time, invest in a good cooler bag, and carry it everywhere. Just make sure not to keep any trigger foods around (the two to three foods that you have low control over and which you tend to eat in large quantities). Even if they are healthy, if you can't control yourself around them, don't keep them in easy access.

REASON #13: Being inconsistent – Sticking to your meal plan for one week and then not the next, or just on weekdays is not being consistent. Being 60% compliant is not going to propel you toward your weight or fat-loss goals. It's like taking two steps forward and one step back. I personally like to apply something I call the 80% rule (or 90% if fat-loss is your goal), which means that you eat on track 80% of the time, and leave 20% room for eating off-plan.

REASON #14: Making excuses – People have stressful days all the time, and bad things will happen throughout our lives. Sticking to your plan throughout a difficult or trying time will allow you to handle the situation better. If you are healthy and strong, you will react better, provide better support, sleep better, have more energy, and generally better withstand stress.

REASON #15: Giving up too early – Most of us are conditioned to seek immediate gratification. Sometimes clients are making huge improvements, but because those improvements may be too small to the naked eye, they give up when they are right around the corner from a huge break-through. It took time for your body to get in the shape it is in now; give it time to get in the shape you desire as well. Two weeks is not enough to see massive physical improvements in your body. Instead, focus on the other improvements you are making in the meantime (see next point).

REASON #16: Relying too much on the scale – If you are looking for success solely by the numbers you see on a scale (weight, body fat, or otherwise), you are setting yourself up for disappointment. The scale is only one measure of success. That is why it's important to track more than one variable throughout your weight or fat loss journey. At our bi-weekly check-ins, my clients track their progress in several ways: they take comparison photos, provide anthropometric measurements, measure strength and cardiovascular improvements, measure fat mass and muscle mass, track energy levels and sleep quality, assess the way their clothes fit, etc. There is no better way to kill your motivation than relying on one measure alone.

REASON #17: Not drinking enough water – This is an oldie but a biggie. If you don't drink enough water, you may think you are hungry when you are actually thirsty, not to mention that if you are dehydrated, your metabolism can drop by up to 2%[21]. Being dehydrated can also make you tired and diminish your performance in the gym, which means you won't be able to work at the intensity you need to in order to make improvements.

REASON #18: Putting yourself last – Being a martyr never helps anyone. If you don't take time to focus on your health now (think of it as preventative medicine), once you get sick, it's too late. It's a lot easier to prevent diabetes and heart disease than it is to heal from it. Make time for your meal preparation and your workouts. Let your family and friends know it's a priority for you to get healthy. Better yet, involve them in your plans.

REASON #19: Sitting too much – This is huge. We sit too much these days (an average of ten hours a day). Even if you spend an hour exercising, it cannot make up for those 10 hours of inactivity every day. Break up those long bouts of sitting with a few minutes of movement to bring your metabolism back up. Turn off your computer, turn off the TV, turn off the video games, and get outside and move around. If you find it hard to get motivated, buy a pedometer (or use the app on your cell phone), and aim to get in 10,000 steps a day[22].

REASON #20: Thinking you're not worthy – Ah, self-sabotage, it's a wonderful thing. This is probably the #1 reason why people think they do everything right and yet can't lose weight. Negative self-talk ("I'm so fat") and using negative language ("It's impossible") will get you nowhere. As Henry Ford said, "Whether you think you can, or you think you can't, you're right.[23]" So delve deep, believe you're worth it, and change that attitude around.

How to navigate social events

One area that many of my clients struggle with on their path to wellness is how to navigate social events. Inevitably it's that time of year for socializing again (hello, winter, spring, summer, and fall) and you are trying your best to avoid the types of foods and drinks that are par for course at these types of events. With temptation lurking around every corner, is your only option to turn into a social pariah? Since we know that's not reality, you at least need to be prepared to face some of your toughest times around the holidays.

With parties in full swing, and all your family and friends throwing caution to the wind and indulging left and right, is it possible to resist eating the types of food that you know will add inches to your waistline, shut down your immune system, and make you sluggish for days? Well, with a few simple strategies and some advanced planning, you can learn how to keep your health and wellness at the top of your mental priority list and emerge having taken one step ahead instead of one step back:

1. Motivate yourself by writing down the reasons you started a new lifestyle in the first place. This is your *why*. Know your *why*. Remember it, or even better, pull it out and re-read it every time you feel temptation beckoning.

2. Start the day off with a healthy balanced breakfast consisting of protein, vegetables, and some healthy fat. This will ensure that your blood-sugar levels are balanced, and you will be less likely to feel famished later in the day.

3. Eat a small snack consisting of protein, fibre, and fat before you leave for a social event. A small snack will ensure that you are not starving by the time the food arrives, and it will still leave you enough room to participate in the festivities.

4. If you are going out to eat with friends, recommend a restaurant that has healthy

options. Take time to look at the menu online beforehand and choose your entrée ahead of time. Another option is to split an entrée with a friend or ask the waiter to only bring you half a serving.

5.   Don't hang around the buffet table; if the food is not within eyesight, you can't be tempted by it. Focus on enjoying the company instead, and make sure you have some sparkling water to sip on to keep your hands occupied.

6.   Don't drink on an empty stomach. Stick to water or mineral water until after your meal. Remember that alcohol reduces your inhibitions and clouds your judgement, interfering with your ability to make sound decisions. Also, try to stick to lower-calorie options like wine and vodka sodas.

7.   When you do eat, eat sitting down, and take your time to savour and chew every bite. It is much more difficult to overeat (or to eat the wrong thing) if you are present and mindful.

8.   Plan out your meal before you dig in. As soon as the food is served, mentally note what foods / dishes you will be eating before you indulge, and stick to your plan.

9.   Try not to overdo it at social events. This is especially true if you have a very healthy social life. Stick to your guns on this one, because inevitably, by the time you realize how much you were eating while being distracted you will have eaten much more than what your stomach can comfortably store at any one time.

10.   Stop being apologetic for making healthier choices. Own your choices, stand up for them, and act as if you are happy about it, even if you are not. Remember, other people's opinions are none of your business.

11.   To prevent your host from encouraging you to eat more or indulge in foods that don't fit into your plan, pull your host aside ahead of time, and explain your situation. That way he or she will be less likely to push you to eat more food or place extra servings onto your plate without your consent.

12.   Take a break if things become too overwhelming and you feel your willpower wavering. Grab a friend and head outside to take a walk or just move to another room where food is not tempting you at every turn.

13.   Remember that you are doing yourself and your body a favour by abstaining from foods that are full of empty calories and devoid of nutrients. Familiarizing yourself with the ingredients in the foods you will be eating helps a lot. Once you know what's in your food, you can't un-know...and it becomes harder to make poor decisions.

14.   Keep the focus on the social aspect of the festivities, not on the food. You are there to see your friends, have fun, and catch up — so do exactly that!

15.   Keep in mind that every time you give in to temptation, you are not just feeding yourself unhealthy food, but you are also feeding an unhealthy HABIT. Every time you give

in to temptation, you are weakening your resolve, making it easier for yourself to give in again and again and again....

16.   That being said, allow yourself to indulge once in a while, but plan it out ahead of time. Set a limit and stick to it, unless you are an all-or-nothing person. In that case, sticking to nothing is better, until you can learn to live in moderation.

17.   Ensure that you plan an intense resistance training or HIIT workout prior to your social event. At least you'll arrive knowing your workout for the day has been done and the calories are more likely to be used for rebuilding and repairing your muscle tissue than for accumulating more fat stores.

18.   Instead of always planning social events around food, suggest a healthier social event that centers on being active; go to the beach, hit the slopes, go for a hike, etc.

19.   Another option is to offer to host. You can serve a healthier menu and provide guests with the recipes to your new healthy dishes, or suggest a salad / fruit bar where every guest brings one salad / fruit bar ingredient and everyone can make their own salad.

20.   Finally, remember that balance is important, but — if you are reading this — you have likely already had a LOT of experience INDULGING for the past few years, so remember, now is the time to swing the pendulum in the other direction and show a bit more moderation.

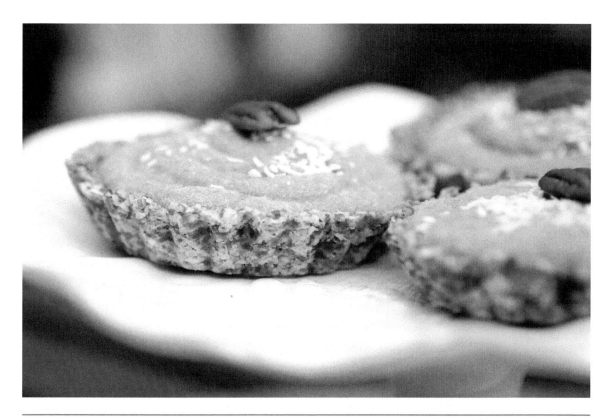

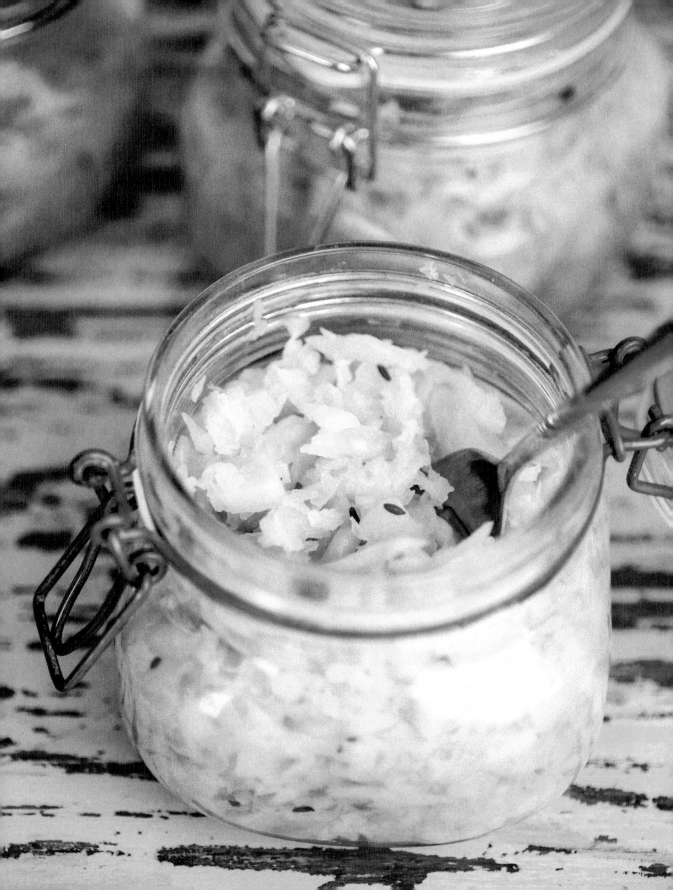

SETTING UP YOUR KITCHEN FOR SUCCESS

Prepping Your Kitchen

We already spoke about setting up your environment for success and your kitchen set-up is a large part of that. Whether you are just embarking on your wellness journey or whether you have just taken too many detours lately, it's a good idea to start with a clean slate. So, in order to make room for all of the healthy grocery shopping and the healthy cooking that you will be doing, you will need to make room in your pantry, fridge and freezer.

First start off by getting rid of all the junk food (high-calorie, low-nutrient content foods) that you have accumulated as well as any trigger foods that you have lying around. If you feel that you might get a big uproar from your family members (although it's good to bear in mind that you are doing this for them too) then at least take these nutrient-void foods and store them some place out of reach (like in a box in your basement) so it becomes less convenient to reach for them.

Next, throw out anything that has sugar listed in the first three ingredients (and likely multiple times thereafter). Remember that sugar can come in many different forms and has many different names, so you need to inform yourself and become a bit of a detective. For example, sugar can also be called corn syrup, cane sugar, fruit juice concentrate, dextrose, fructose, molasses, maple syrup, agave nectar, lactose, maltose, and sucrose (and anything else ending in –ose), just to name a few. There are in fact at least 50 different names of sugar[24] that I know of, and although some of these sugars are natural or less processed than regular table sugar, it does not mean that they are a healthier choice (especially if it has three forms of sugar). Check out www.michellevodrazka.com/sugar-saboteurs for the full list.

Finally, make sure to toss any items that you never use or that are way past their best before date. These items are just taking up space in your kitchen (and your life) adding to the clutter and holding you back from moving forward. While you are at it, take some extra time to clean out your cabinets and drawers and give away or throw out anything that you aren't using regularly. Having a clean, well-organized kitchen will increase the likelihood that you enjoy being in the one room that is the greatest predictor of a healthy life.

It All Starts at the Grocery Store

I have a love/hate relationship with grocery shopping. I love it because it's where healthy eating starts, and I hate it because the food industry has made it incredibly confusing and difficult to make good food choices. Stocking your fridge, freezer, and pantry with healthy choices will make you much more likely to achieve your health, nutrition, and fitness goals, because you are creating an environment for success. So, if you exercise your willpower in the store, you won't need to exercise willpower at home and it becomes much easier to follow through on your good intentions. Here are a few tips to help you get started and to guide you through your next grocery adventure:

1. First of all, where you shop matters. Supporting your local farmers not only ensures that you get super-fresh, seasonal produce, but you also will know exactly where your food is coming from and how it was grown and harvested. Local farmers often sell their goods at farmers' markets, at roadside stands, and via food delivery programs and community-supported agriculture shares (CSAs). I highly encourage you to get to know your local farmers and to take advantage of fresh, local foods. If you don't have this option, shopping at a farm-fresh market, a local health-food store, or health-focused grocery stores like Whole Foods or Farm Boy are your next best option. Choose local and organic first, local second, organic third, and conventional last.

2. Remember, if you don't bring the junk home, you can't be tempted by it. If you want to treat yourself, save it for a special occasion and then go out and buy a single serving and savour every bite. Or better yet, when a craving strikes, write down the food or meal that you are craving and save it for a weekend treat. Remember, treat is defined as something saved for a special occasion that causes special pleasure or delight; it is not meant to be a regular occurrence. Unfortunately, in our society, we have gotten so used to seeking instant gratification that we now indulge multiple times a day and think nothing of it! No wonder 2/3 of our population is overweight or obese.[25]

3. Now, we already discussed this, but the adage is true and it's absolutely worth repeating: If it's made in a factory and comes in a box, chances are, it's not good for you. Note that there are some exceptions to this, but if it has a long list of ingredients that you cannot pronounce, it definitely belongs in the trash, and not in your body. Stick to whole, fresh, single-ingredient foods, and when you do buy foods that come in packages, make sure to read your labels very carefully.

4. Read the ingredient list on the back of the label that lists, in descending order of prominence, all of the ingredients in the food item. This is where you can make informed decisions and identify any hidden ingredients, like sugars, allergens, preservatives, additives, trans-fats and salts. For example, if you pick up almost any of the major cereals on the market today, you'll notice that either the first or the second ingredient listed is sugar. Add to that wheat, salt, another form of sugar, a bit of food coloring, some more sugar (in another form), a few preservatives, and to balance it all out, a sprinkle of artificial flavour, and you get the "delicious" food that you have just eaten, all under the banner of "a nutritious breakfast". Unfortunately, the only nutritious food you actually ate were the berries that you (hopefully) added on top of your cereal. Yikes!

5. Make a grocery list and stick to it. To assist you in making healthy choices, later in this chapter, I have provided you with a list of foods that I fill my fridge with, which you can use as a guide the next time you go to the grocery store. Every one of the foods on the list will give you a lot of bang for your buck and will provide you with the nutritional support you need to start creating a well-balanced, solid nutritional base, which is a requirement for a healthy metabolism. So, the next time you go shopping, remember to fill up your cart with

all those nutritiously rich foods that I've included on the list — and, just for fun, while you are standing in line, sneak a peek at other people's grocery carts. I guarantee you will be shocked at what you see and incredibly proud of the choices that you have just made.

6.   If it's not good for you, it certainly isn't good for the kids. Your children do not need junk food, so don't bring it home "for them". You are the most important role model in your child's life. If you keep healthy food in the house, make healthy choices, and indulge only on occasion, they will learn from your example. Feeding your kids junk food regularly or having it too readily available will only lead to poor food choices, tooth decay, mood swings, erratic energy levels, obesity, and a lack of proper nutritional support for their growing bodies. Jamie Oliver, of the Food Revolution, gives an incredibly compelling speech about nutrition, the obesity epidemic and children's long term health at www.ted.com/talks/ jamie_oliver.html.[26]

7.   Similarly, try not to resort to using junk food or sweets as a reward, neither for your kids nor for yourself, as it sends the message that these foods are more valuable than other foods. Furthermore, research has shown that the more frequently that parents use food as a reward or punishment, the more likely it is that they will grow into adults who eat in the absence of hunger (i.e. they may resort to eating when they are feeling down or when they had a bad day). So why not find other ways to reward yourself and your kids? Take the kids to the park, make a craft with them or treat yourself to the spa or a nice bath.

Stocking a Real Food Kitchen

In order to make your transition to a healthy lifestyle a little bit easier, here is a list of foods that you will generally find in my kitchen. Please notice that I do not use non-fat foods or foods with artificial sweeteners. I personally believe that we all need some healthy fat in our diets and that substituting real fat by adding sugar or chemicals is not the way to go. In fact, dietary restrictions on fats are being dropped in the forthcoming *2015 Dietary Guidelines for Americans*.[27] which is a huge step in the right direction.

I also believe in stocking my kitchen with foods that are as close as possible to the way nature intended them and that is primarily what you will find on my healthy shopping list. This list is also available for download on my website www.michellevodrazka.com/healthy-shopping-list. Although I have done my best to be as comprehensive as possible, please do not consider this an exhaustive list.

Now if you are ready for a real overhaul, and are looking for a hands-on, practical, step-by-step course on how to properly stock a real food kitchen, check out Meghan Telpner's amazing workshop at www.meghantelpner.com/undiet-meal-prep-made-easy-workshop. Although I provide some general advice on meal prep later in this chapter, it is nowhere near as extensive as what Meghan covers in her course, which includes 21 instructional videos and 40 PDF documents on topics such as exactly how to store dry goods and produce for optimal freshness and step-by-step information on how to batch cook. I took this course myself when I started to dive into culinary nutrition and I learned so much!

FRIDGE:

- fresh herbs (basil, thyme, mint, oregano, parsley, cilantro, rosemary, etc.)

- fresh organic chicken, fish, or grass-fed beef

- nut and seed milks (hemp, almond, Brazil nut, sesame, coconut, etc.)

- gluten-free tortillas and gluten-free sprouted bread

- organic, full-fat coconut milk (I like Earth's Choice organic coconut milk)

- grass-fed ghee

- fresh veggies (broccoli, cauliflower, carrots, mini tomatoes, sweet bell peppers, mushrooms, zucchini, spinach, squash, beets, cucumbers, asparagus, green beans, celery, leeks, collard greens, kale, etc.)

- fresh fruit (blueberries, raspberries, strawberries, kiwis, apples, cantaloupe, avocados, oranges, lemons, cranberries, grapefruit, pears, red grapes, pineapples, etc.)

- organic eggs

- marinated vegetables (artichokes, olives, red peppers, etc.)

- omega-3 rich nuts and seeds (walnuts, flax seeds, etc.)

- healthy, unrefined oils (flaxseed, hempseed, walnut, etc.)

- organic hot sauce

- organic tamari sauce

- liquid aminos (I like Bragg Liquid Aminos)

- healthy or homemade salad dressings (again, Bragg has some great ones)

- homemade hummus

- real maple syrup

- Dijon mustard

- homemade pesto

- water (infused water, mineral water, etc.)

- kombucha (I like RISE kombucha)

- organic coffee beans

- gluten-free greens powder (I like Genuine Health Greens+ O powder)

FREEZER:

- organic boneless, skinless chicken breasts

- whole organic chickens

- fatty fish (salmon, sardines, mackerel, rainbow trout, herring, etc.)

- white fish (striped bass, pollock, sole, flounder, haddock, tilapia, etc.)

- shellfish (oysters, shrimp, scallops, etc.)

- grass-fed, ground meats (turkey, chicken, beef, etc.)

- wild game (bison, venison, elk, wild boar, etc.)

- organic grass-fed beef bones

- homemade stock (chicken, beef, vegetable, etc.)

- homemade soups and leftovers

- frozen veggies (broccoli, peas, green beans, cauliflower, carrots, etc.)

- frozen greens (spinach, kale, collards, Swiss chard, etc.)

- frozen edamame

- frozen fruit (berries, pineapple, peaches, papaya, mango, bananas, etc.)

- frozen spices (cilantro, basil, parsley, garlic, mint, dill, etc.)

- gluten-free tortillas

- gluten-free sprouted bread

PANTRY:

- whole-grain, gluten-free pasta (brown rice, buckwheat, quinoa, etc.)

- gluten-free oats (oat groats, steel-cut oats, rolled oats, etc.)

- gluten-free grains (quinoa, amaranth, millet, buckwheat, rice, etc.)

- rice wraps

- gluten-free flours (almond, oat, brown rice, quinoa, buckwheat, arrowroot, etc.)

- root vegetables (potatoes, sweet potatoes, yams, beets, turnips, squash, rutabaga, onions, garlic, ginger, turmeric, etc.)

- dried organic herbs and spices (basil, oregano, nutmeg, cayenne pepper, thyme, rosemary, turmeric, cinnamon, cumin, parsley, marjoram, coriander, curry, paprika, cloves, ginger, caraway seeds, Italian seasoning, garlic powder, Herbamare, etc.)

- sea salt (Celtic, Himalayan, etc.)

- organic, BPA-free canned beans (chickpeas, black beans, lentils, pinto, cannellini, etc.)

- dried beans (chickpeas, black beans, lentils, kidney beans, split peas, etc.)

- healthy, unrefined oils (olive oil, coconut oil, avocado oil, sesame oil, etc.)

- vinegars (Bragg Apple Cider Vinegar, balsamic vinegar, white wine vinegar, etc.)

- organic, BPA-free canned coconut milk (I like Earth's Choice organic coconut milk)

- organic applesauce

- organic, BPA-free canned pumpkin

- organic teas (rooibos, green tea, chamomile, ginger, mint, licorice, oat straw, etc.)

- caffeine-free coffee substitute (I like Dandy Blend)

- organic salsa (I like Neal Brothers organic salsa)

- organic tomato and pasta sauce (again, I like Neal Brothers organic pasta sauce)

- organic, BPA-free canned tomato paste

- organic, BPA-free canned tomatoes

- organic, BPA-free canned fish (Albacore tuna, sardines, sockeye salmon, mackerel, etc.)

PANTRY:

- organic stock (chicken, vegetable, beef, etc.)

- 70% dark chocolate (I like Giddy Yoyo's organic chocolate)

- dairy-free chocolate chips or carob chips (I like Enjoy Life dairy-free chocolate chips)

- raw cacao powder (I like Navitas Naturals raw cacao powder)

- raw cacao nibs (again, I like Navitas Naturals cacao nibs)

- baking cocoa (I buy mine at Costco)

- seeds (chia, hemp, pumpkin, sunflower, etc.)

- nuts (almonds, cashews, pecans, Brazil nuts, hazelnuts, etc.)

- dried, shredded, unsweetened coconut

- dried organic fruit (cranberries, raisins, dates, mulberries, goji berries, cherries, figs, etc.)

- natural nut and seed butters (almond, cashew, tahini, sunflower seed, etc.)

- natural sweeteners (coconut palm sugar, raw honey, sucanat, blackstrap molasses, etc.)

- organic popcorn kernels

- nutritional yeast (I like Bragg Nutritional Yeast Seasoning)

- aluminum-free baking powder

- organic baking soda

- vanilla beans

- pure extracts (pure vanilla extract, pure mint extract)

- sea vegetables and seaweed (dulse, nori, kelp, kombu, nori, arame, etc.)

- dried mushrooms or mushroom powder (shiitake, chaga, turkey tails, reishi, etc.)

- grass-fed gelatin (I like Great Lakes gelatin)

- vegan protein powders (I like Genuine Health Fermented Vegan Proteins+ powder)

- other supplements (vitamins, minerals, digestive enzymes, herbs, etc.)

Why Labels (and Calories) Deceive Us

The first thing you need to know is that label reading when grocery shopping is vital, but labels are also incredibly deceiving. Here's why. There are two distinct food label areas on packaged foods. One area is usually found on the back of the package or container and includes the nutrition facts table and the list of ingredients. The other one is usually on the front side of the package or container and includes health claims like "fat-free", "all-natural", and "heart-healthy". Unfortunately, the front of the package is really just marketing "real estate" and is there for the sole purpose of helping food marketers sell as many products as possible.

In my opinion, even the nutrition facts table on the back of the package has very limited value, for a number of reasons. First of all, the entire table is based on the premise that counting calories and artificially tracking nutrients is beneficial, or that it's useful for making healthier choices or achieving overall health, which it's not. All that measuring and counting using databases, apps or software is super complicated and riddled with error. Our diets used to be way healthier, and we were able to make healthy choices for ourselves and our families without complicated calculations and government guidelines.

Now, that's not to say that we can't benefit from the advances that we have made in nutritional research, but the fact is that if we would just return to eating the way we used to before the industrial revolution — when the bulk of our diets consisted of whatever fresh produce we could get locally, seasonally, and organically — then we would not need to painstakingly count calories or nutrients to maintain our health.

Furthermore, when we rely on counting calories or nutrients, we feel comforted by the fact that we have accurate information, but the reality is that we don't. According to Precision Nutrition, research has shown that calorie counts can be off by up to 25% due to incorrect labeling, laboratory measurement errors, and food quality[28]. Then, on top of that, estimating the calories we consume can also be off by up to 25% because of the equipment or tool that you are using to measure calories (think for example of MyFitnessPal, which allows users to enter calorie and nutrient information into MyFitnessPal's database, which may be completely unreliable), individual differences in food (for example, there are huge variances in the size of an average apple), and user error (for example, making mistakes in assessing correct serving size and under-estimating the amount of food consumed).[28]

The other drawback to counting calories is that it shifts our focus from the quality of our food to the quantity of our food. We lose sight of the fact that our food truly is our medicine. If you feed yourself with 2,000 calories worth of nutrient-void junk foods, it will hurt your body rather than heal it. Although the energy value (calorie count) may be the same, nutrient-dense foods will yield an infinitely higher amount of energy than nutrient-void foods, which will drain you of energy. Another way to think of it is that over-processed, nutrient-void foods (which usually come in boxes, containers, or packages) are 'dead' foods, and don't provide your body with the "living" components of food that are needed to keep it alive, vital, and thriving.

As mentioned previously, the only part of a food label that is worth the paper it's printed on, is the ingredient list. This is where you can find out whether the food (or food-like product) is supporting your health, or compromising it. Here are ten general suggestions for selecting foods and decoding food labels:

1.   Plan ahead by bringing a grocery list and try not to shop hungry. That way you will be less likely to be tempted by spur-of-the-moment purchases or powerful food marketing.

2.   Buy as many single ingredient foods as possible — like those that don't need labels.

3.   Remember to ignore the information on the front of the label - it's just marketing real estate. Flip that puppy over and start reading the ingredient list.

4.   The shorter the ingredient list, the better: seven ingredients or less is best.

5.   Don't buy a food if you can't pronounce the ingredients or if you don't know what they are. At the very least, use your cellphone to look them up before you put them in your body!

6.   Avoid foods that have sugar listed as one of the top three ingredients, or that list sugar multiple times, under different names.

7.   Don't buy foods that have packages that appeal to kids (think bright colors and cartoon characters) or that try really hard to convince you how healthy they are (this is called health-washing and is a really shoddy practice in the food industry).

8.   Try your best to avoid food ingredients that have been linked to adverse health effects or implicated in allergic reactions, such as Monosodium Glutamate (MSG), High Fructose Corn Syrup (HFCS), and hydrogenated or trans fats, among others. For more information on what ingredients to avoid, see my *Top Nine Worst Food Ingredients* list.

9.   Buy organic when possible. This will ensure that the contents of your food are at 95% free of pesticides, herbicides, fungicides, insecticides, artificial food additives, and dyes, and that they are free of genetic modification. Check the Dirty Dozen™ list later in this chapter.

10.   Finally, if it doesn't look like food you could find in nature or that you could make yourself at home, leave it on the shelf.

It's insane what types of ingredients are allowed into our food nowadays. Chemicals, additives, preservatives and stabilizers are not meant to be ingested! They certainly aren't doing us any favours and in fact, could be doing us harm, so why take a chance with your health? Although some of these ingredients have been deemed to be safe for human consumption in small amounts, it all adds up over the span of a lifetime.

I personally make an effort to eat as fresh as possible in order to minimize ingredients such as these, but that's not always realistic, so I at least try to avoid the worst offenders, which you can find on the next page. Now, unfortunately, this is by no means an exhaustive list, so I encourage you to do more research and learn what is in your food. Don't assume that it is safe or good for you just because it is on our grocery store shelves.

Top Nine Worst Food Ingredients

Food Ingredient	Found in	Used	Avoid because
Trans fats and partially hydrogenated vegetable oils	Commercial baked goods, crackers, cookies, margarine, salad dressings, and chips	As a fat that increases shelf life and stabilizes flavour	They boost LDL, lower HDL, and are linked to heart disease, diabetes, and cellular degradation.[29]
High Fructose Corn Syrup (HFCS)	Soft drinks, salad dressings, sauces, breakfast cereals, bars, and breads	As a sweetener	It increases the risk of diabetes and metabolic syndrome.[30]
Artificial sweeteners like sucralose (Splenda), aspartame (Equal), saccharine (Sweet n Low), and Acesulfame-K (Sweet One)	In foods labeled sugar-free like diet soda, gum, and many popular sports supplements	As a sweetener	They are associated with obesity, and they affect healthy gut bacteria.[31]
Monosodium Glutamate (MSG) (E621)	Canned foods, soups, salad dressings, chips, and packaged sausages	As a flavour enhancer	Linked to fatty liver disease and obesity.[32]
Butylated Hydroxyl-Anisole (E320), BHA, and BHT	Cereals, breads, chips, crackers, gum, and snack foods	As preservatives in high-fat foods to keep them from going rancid	BHA and BHT may be human carcinogens. They disrupt proper hormone production.[33]

Top Nine Worst Food Ingredients

Food Ingredient	Found in	Used	Avoid because
Sodium nitrite (E250) and sodium nitrate (E251)	Jerky, bacon, luncheon meats, sausages, hot dogs, and smoked meats	As a preservative	They are associated with headaches, nausea, rashes, and vomiting in sensitive individuals, and are linked to oral, stomach, brain, bladder, and pancreatic cancers.[34]
Benzoic acid (E210) and sodium benzoate (E211)	Salad dressings, sauces, jams, carbonated drinks, pickles and condiments	As a preservative	They can produce the carcinogen benzene and have been linked to cellular changes.[35]
Sodium sulphite	Wine and dried fruit	As a preservative	It is linked to asthma, breathing problems, headaches, and rashes.[36]
Food colourings like brilliant blue (E133), erythrosine (E127) FD&C red No. 3, and tartrazine (E102) FD&C yellow No. 5	Candy, gum, ice cream, popsicles, cereals, and cake icing	To enhance the colour of food	They are linked to ADHD, adverse allergic reactions, and cancer.[37]

Is Buying Organic Really Necessary?

In an ideal world, all the food available to everybody would be organic, with no artificial pesticides, fertilizers, antibiotics, or growth hormones, and it would be free of Genetically Modified Organisms (GMOs), produced using sustainable practices — and inexpensive. Unfortunately, that scenario is not even close to our current reality. When we go grocery shopping at regular supermarkets, most of the produce and fresh animal products we find are conventionally farmed and raised. Conventional farming is, in today's day and age, quite the opposite of organic farming.

According to the US Department of Agriculture, among other characteristics, conventional farming systems extensively use pesticides, fertilizers, and external energy inputs; depend on agribusiness; and grow single / row crops continuously over many seasons[38]. These practices exhaust soil nutrition (resulting in plants with less nutrients), wipe out the natural micro-organism equilibrium of the soil (and the ability for the soil to protect itself, and plants, naturally against disease and pests), and leave the plant with a toxic load of chemicals (which we ideally don't want to ingest).

For example, if you take a look at www.whatsonmyfood.org, run by the Pesticide Action Network, you will see that conventionally-grown apples have 47 different pesticide residues, blueberries have 57 different pesticide residues, and peaches have 62 different pesticide residues, as documented by the USDA. In fact, the website even lists exactly what each of the pesticides are. I don't know about you, but I have no desire to ingest this many different types of pesticides on a regular basis!

The bad news is that the cost of switching over completely from conventional to organic is just not something that most of us can afford. The good news is that there are certain fruits and vegetables that contain very low levels of pesticide residues. For example, avocados test positive for one pesticide residue and pineapples test positive for six. But how do you know which ones are safe(r) to buy conventionally and which ones you absolutely need to buy organic?

This is where I introduce you to an incredible list created by the wonderful people at the Environmental Working Group (EWG, www.ewg.org)[39]. Each year, they rate conventional produce in the US according to the level of pesticide residue (tested once the produce reaches the grocers' shelves). The produce with the highest pesticide load makes it onto a list called the Dirty Dozen™ and the produce with the lowest pesticide load makes it onto a list called the Clean Fifteen™. You can find the list for 2015[40] on the next page.

Besides shopping according to this list, you can also reach out to your local farmers. Even though they may not be certified organic (because it costs money to get certified) some of them don't use pesticides. Visiting a local farmers market, or calling farmers in your community are the best ways to find out this information. Plus, by choosing to shop locally, you support your local community and your produce will be freshly picked, which means they will automatically be higher in nutrients than if you were to buy them imported from other countries or grown on farms hundreds, or thousands, of miles away.

Dirty Dozen ™

Apples

Celery

Cherry Tomatoes

Cucumbers

Grapes

Nectarines

Peaches

Potatoes

Snap Peas

Spinach

Strawberries

Sweet Bell Peppers

+ Hot Peppers

+ Collard Greens

Clean Fifteen ™

Asparagus

Avocados

Cabbage

Cantaloupe

Cauliflower

Eggplant

Grapefruit

Kiwi

Mangoes

Onions

Papayas

Pineapples

Sweet Corn

Sweet Peas (frozen)

Now, while we're on the topic of toxic chemicals, I also want to point out that the EWG has numerous other incredible resources on its site such as the *Skin Deep Guide to Cosmetics*[41], and the *Guide to Healthy Cleaning*[42]. These are two excellent guides that can help you reduce your overall chemical use and lower your body's toxic load. I highly recommend that you check them out.

Kitchen Tools for Success

Now it's time to get to business. In order to make your kitchen adventures fun instead of frustrating, and easy instead of elusive, you need the right kitchen tools. Having the right tools can make food prep much easier and faster, making time spent in the kitchen more enjoyable. I personally spend a lot of time in my kitchen anyway, but it's by choice, and I know it's not everyone else's idea of a fabulous time. So, I have compiled a list of the kitchen tools that I use most often, and which have become invaluable to me. Keep in mind that when I first started, I only had the basics. A well-stocked kitchen takes time to build, so work your way up to it at your own pace. But remember, the chef of the family is the doctor of the family. So if you want to invest in your health, here are the tools that can help you do it:

1. **Food processor** – This is undoubtedly the kitchen tool that I use the most. I'll tell you why: I cheat in the kitchen. Yes, it's true. With four kids and two jobs, finding ways to cheat (make things as quick and simple as possible) is critical to my kitchen success. I even thought about writing an entire cookbook full of recipes that only required a food processor — maybe I still will. Anyway, a good food processor, like a KitchenAid, can chop vegetables, shred cheese, chop nuts, mix cookie dough, make hummus, and even turn bananas into the most delicious soft-serve ice cream. A food processor does a lot to quicken your food prep; basically, anything that needs to be chopped or mixed can be done in a food processor. A good food processor will run you about $150–200 but is truly invaluable.

2. **Blender** – I primarily use my blender for making smoothies or puréeing soups, but if you have a really good blender like a Vitamix or a Blendtec, you can also use it in much the same way you would use your food processor. In addition to soups and smoothies, you can make sauces, ice cream, salad dressings, hummus, and more. A Vitamix will run you close to $600 and a Blendtec close to $400. I personally own a Vitamix, which I adore, and to this day, I have not met anyone who has regretted their purchase. I know this may seem like an exorbitant price for a blender, but the fact is that this machine is so incredibly well put together that it will last you many, many years. If you really cannot afford spending this much money on a kitchen appliance, you might want to consider a Nutribullet, which can be purchased for around $100 and with which a lot of my clients are quite happy.

3. **Immersion blender** – An immersion blender, also called a stick blender or a hand blender, is used to purée food in the container in which it is prepared. I love my immersion blender, but I really only use it for puréeing soups (which in my household occurs about two to three times per week, because my kids won't eat any soups with "chunks" in them). However, you can also use it for emulsifying sauces. An average immersion blender costs anywhere from around $40–$100.

4. **Stand mixer** – It took me many years before I finally invested in a stand mixer. I used a hand-held version for many years, in part due to cost but also due to counter space. Whether or not it is worth investing in, depends on the mixing capacity that you need. I found that eventually a hand-held mixer was not able to thoroughly mix the batters I was making, and so I upgraded to a KitchenAid stand mixer. A hand-held mixer can be purchased pretty inexpensively ($30–$80), whereas a stand mixer will generally run you around $200–$400.

5. **Juicer** – There are two main types of juicers, centrifugal juicers and masticating juicers. I personally prefer to use a masticating juicer, because it retains more nutrients, and is quieter, more efficient, and more versatile. The drawback is that a masticating juicer can cost quite a bit more than a centrifugal juicer, and will run you around $300–$500.

Here are some other basic kitchen tools that I recommend:

large, medium and small pot	good cast-iron frying pan
ceramic green pan	glass baking pans of varying sizes
muffin pan	silicone muffin cups
large stainless steel baking sheet	good set of knives
different sized mixing bowls	zester
coffee/nut grinder	garlic press
rolling pin	ice cream scoop (trust me)
sieve	colander
spatula	citrus juicer
can opener	milk frother
potato masher	coffee maker
peeler	grater
whisk	spiralizer
measuring cups and spoons	good set of cutting boards
wooden spoons	glass containers for food storage
mason jars of all sizes	nut milk bag

Master the Art of Meal Prep

I love cooking and am happy to spend hours in the kitchen experimenting with different techniques and food combinations, but I know most people don't share my excitement for the kitchen. I also know what it feels like to be hungry and tired and pressed for time. When this happens, most of us are tempted to cut corners to get food on the table - stat! We buy ready-to-eat food, go to a restaurant, or order take-out. Don't get me wrong: it's not the end of the world if we do this on occasion and in balance with eating mainly homemade meals. The problems occur when relying on what's convenient becomes the rule rather than the exception.

When someone else prepares our food, especially when it's mass-produced, we lose control over what's in it. In order to make mass-produced food taste as good as freshly-prepared, homemade food, it is usually loaded with salt, sugar and fat, along with a ton of preservatives. We end up missing out on the vitamins, minerals, antioxidants, and phytonutrients we need, which can set us up for increased hunger, unbalanced hormones, elevated blood sugar levels, low energy, and poor performance. Plus, it can get really expensive to eat out regularly.

So here I am, to rescue you, and show you that there's a trick to having awesome, homemade meals in minimal time. You just need a little bit of organization! Proper meal preparation is the secret to optimizing your time in the kitchen. I have broken down the process step-by-step, so it's super easy for you to follow. In case you're still skeptical, I'll let you in on a little-known secret – menu and meal prepping is how chefs in restaurants stay on top of things, so this system is proven to work.

All you will need to get started is a bunch of your favorite recipes (or recipe you have been dying to try) and something to write on – this can be good old-fashioned pen and paper, your computer, or even a meal planning app. Ready?

First, we're going to build your menu. You don't have to do this alone. In fact, I suggest that you grab your significant other, your kids, your roommate, or whoever you're going to be sharing meals with, and who may want to have a say in what they get to eat. Start by browsing through some healthy recipes on the internet, leafing through your favorite cookbooks, or pulling out your go-to recipe cards.

Using the *Meal Planning Template* provided, start writing out meal ideas for breakfast, lunch and dinner. I usually suggest keeping breakfast and lunch meals nice and simple by selecting three or four of your favorite recipes, which you can alternate between throughout the week. Allow yourself the option of adding in one on-the-go option for when you are pressed for time, such as a healthy dried fruit and nut bar for breakfast, or a take-out-salad topped with a protein for lunch.

Now it's time to tackle dinner. Dinner is usually the meal that requires the most planning, so being as specific as possible here helps. Pick one recipe for each day of the week. You can even add theme nights if you like, such as 'Meatless Mondays', 'Slow Cooker Tuesdays', 'Kid's Choice', 'Family Favorites', 'Stew Sundays' or simply 'Chicken Night'.

When you are done, print out your meal plan and place it in a binder. Then place hard copies of your chosen recipes into plastic cover sheets (so they don't get dirty when you cook) and add them to the binder behind your meal plan. Voila, your weekly menu is now complete! If you prefer, you can also do this planning online in a word document or with a meal planning app. Over time, you can build up to a month's worth (or more) of weekly menus. That way, no one gets sick of eating the same thing week after week. I also suggest that you try out two to three new recipes each week so you can start to build your repertoire. Toss the recipes that don't work and keep the ones you like for future meal plans. For those of you that are visual learners, here is a sample of a weekly meal plan:

Meal Planning Template

Meal	Ideas/Themes	Recipes
Breakfast	Smoothie Oatmeal Eggs Chia Pudding	Green Goddess Smoothie Cacao Goji Oatmeal Avocado Baked Eggs Peanut Butter Breakfast Pudding
Lunch	Soup & Salad Quinoa Bowl Burger & Veggies	Zucchini Soup & Seeduction Salad Cilantro Quinoa Lime Bowl Nutty Bean Burgers
Dinner	Meatless Monday Taco Tuesday Pasta Wednesday Chicken Thursday Fish Friday Kid's Choice Saturday Stew Sunday	Fresh Quinoa Salad Fish Tacos with Mango Salsa Shrimp in Rosé Sauce Perfect Herb Roasted Chicken Super Simple Asian Salmon Healthy Shepherd's Pie Vegan Sweet Potato Chili

Simple Snack Ideas: Veggies and hummus, an apple with a handful of nuts, a vegan protein shake with berries and ground flax seeds, hard-boiled eggs and veggies, a banana and some nut butter, a handful of homemade trail mix, a few dates filled with pecans, raw veggie sticks and a few olives, a can of sardines with cherry tomatoes, or coconut yogurt with berries

Sticking to a weekly pattern and being organized will increase the likelihood that you will stick to your plan and eat healthier, plus it will also save you time and minimize food waste.

Now, it's time to create a food prep schedule. This is the toughest, most time-consuming, and most rewarding step. Just remember that once this is done, you can re-use it over and over again. Refer to your meal plan, and create a list of tasks that you want to do ahead of time so that when its meal time, the prep is already done and getting ready to eat is a breeze. These tasks could include pre-soaking grains, beans and nuts, washing and chopping food, preparing broths, pre-cooking grains and beans, preparing dressings and healthy snacks, placing ingredients for smoothies in mason jars...you name it! Write down each task, how long it will take, and which day you need to do it. Some people like to separate these tasks into different days, others like to food prep only one day a week. Add your food prep schedule to your binder (or save it online) so everything is in one place.

Once you've built the menu and food prep schedule, it's time to make a shopping list. Review each recipe and list all ingredients you will need along with the quantities you'll need to create each recipe. Cross-reference the list of ingredients with ones you have at home and mark the ones - along with the quantities of each item - that you'll need to buy. Organize your shopping list depending on when you can go shopping and when you plan to prep the dishes. I personally like shopping more frequently so that all ingredients are fresh and food doesn't end up rotting in the fridge, but due to time constraints, some people prefer to make only one large trip to the store each week. I suggest doing whatever works the best for you and your lifestyle.

Now that you have a menu, a food prep schedule, and your groceries, it's time to take action. Remember, whatever you can do in advance is best done in advance, so that building your dish is as fast as possible when it's crunch time. I highly recommend getting the entire family involved in meal prep. Young children can help wash and dry produce and teenagers can help chop and cook simple foods. While you are at it, don't forget to also prep your snacks! Chopping up fresh produce so that it's snack-ready is key in ensuring that you'll make good food choices throughout the day.

I highly suggest pre-dividing all of your snacks for the week into containers so that you can just grab them and go throughout the week. Remember to store everything correctly by refrigerating or freezing it, and try to use non-reactive containers such as stainless steel and glass instead of plastic, which can leech chemicals into your food. Oh, and don't forget to label everything so that you know what's inside each container and how long it will last. I personally meal prep about three times a week, but I also have a large family of six to cook for, so our meals don't last very long. Most of my clients find prepping once or twice a week to be plenty.

Unless you are someone who hates leftovers, I recommend batch cooking, which simply means making extras of everything. Batch cooking will save you a lot of work and time and make your life so much simpler in the long run! A few times a week I cook large batches of rice, quinoa, sweet potatoes, oatmeal, homemade stock, hard-boiled eggs, whole chickens, and beans. I use these throughout the week in various dishes as needed. I also generally re-purpose all of my meals, so if I cook a whole roasted chicken one day, I use the leftover chicken to make an additional two or three meals, like chicken veggie soup, chicken stir fry, or chicken pesto pizzas. Or, I make a huge batch of quinoa and eat it for breakfast as an apple quinoa pudding, for lunch as a few quinoa egg muffins, and for dinner as part of a delicious salad served alongside some salmon.

This process takes time to get used to, and it can seem a bit onerous at first. But as you keep practicing, everything will get easier and faster, and the more you do it, the more efficient you'll become. The best part is that you can reuse the menu, shopping list and meal prep schedule, so once you have a few core menus created, things will be a breeze.

Now that you have a well-stocked fridge, freezer and pantry, and you know how to meal prep properly, all you need to do is to learn how to cook with the fresh, nutritious, whole foods you just bought. So, isn't it handy that you just bought this cookbook? Plus, there are an incredible number of healthy cooking / clean eating and cooking websites and blogs online. You can find entire sites dedicated to gluten-free, dairy-free, nut-free, allergy-friendly, paleo, primal, vegan and vegetarian styles of eating, just to name a few. Don't be afraid to have fun and experiment and use YouTube as a resource for prepping, chopping, and cooking techniques. Involve your family or friends and expect to have a few fails in the kitchen. It's all a part of the learning process which along with a positive attitude, will ultimately lead to a healthier lifestyle.

One Last Thought

I want to leave you with one last thought. I truly believe that each and every one of you is special and beautiful and unique. You are perfect in your imperfections, just as I am. You, like I, are here for a reason, and one of those reasons is to share your unique and special gift with the world, on whatever level that may be. I also believe that we are here to enjoy the miracle of life that surrounds us each and every day. So, I encourage you to pause for a second and recognize that you were born with a gift and that you have the power to build the life that you have always wanted. Until you realize that this choice is yours and that you are the master of your own destiny, things will never change. Life is beautiful. You are beautiful, and each moment is a new opportunity to create a new reality. You are worth investing in yourself. Love yourself. Trust yourself. Treat yourself well. Allow yourself to rise to the occasion and be the best version of yourself that you can be. Everything you think is possible, is possible. You just have to believe it. Now, let's cook!

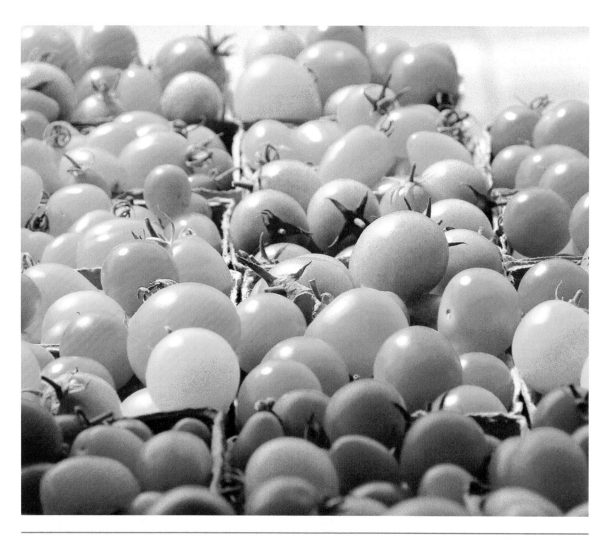

BREAKFASTS

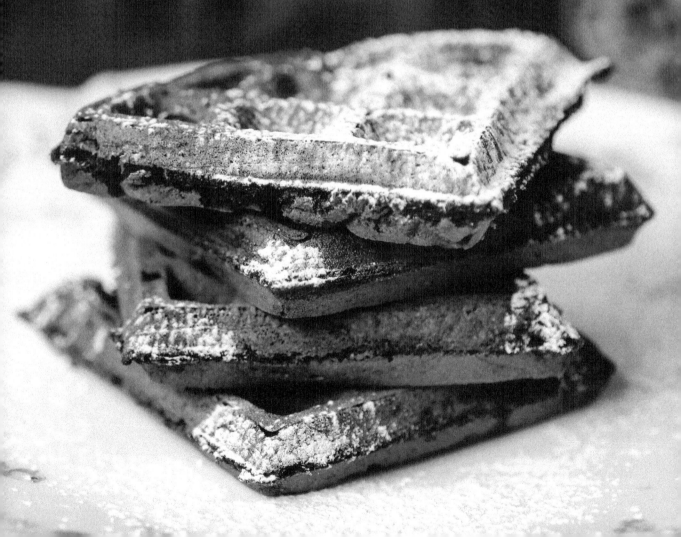

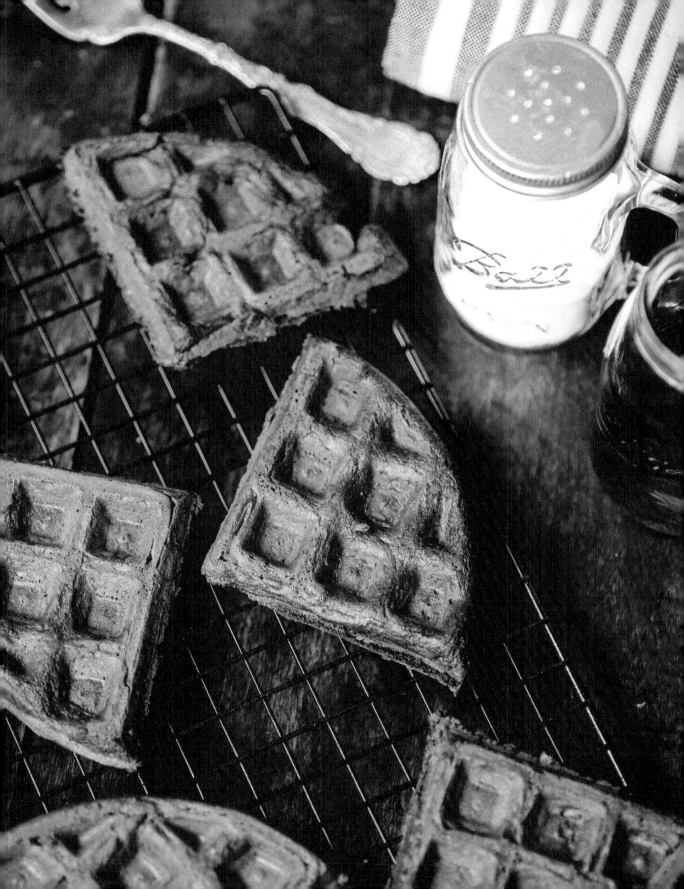

Double Chocolate Chip Waffles

Serves 4–6

Although these waffles sound decadent, they are actually super healthy! Full of whole grains, low in sugar, and high in fibre, these are a great way to start your day, or top them with Chocolate Sauce and Coconut Whipped Cream and serve them for dessert instead.

INGREDIENTS:

- 2 cups nut or seed milk (I use coconut or almond)
- $^1/_2$ cup gluten-free rolled oats
- $^1/_2$ cup brown rice flour
- $^1/_2$ cup buckwheat flour
- $^1/_2$ cup cocoa powder
- $^1/_4$ cup flax meal
- 1 $^1/_2$ teaspoons baking power
- $^1/_2$ teaspoon baking soda
- 1 teaspoon ground cinnamon
- 3 large eggs
- $^1/_4$ cup coconut palm sugar
- 3 tablespoons coconut oil, melted
- 2 teaspoons pure vanilla extract
- optional: $^1/_4$ cup dairy-free chocolate chips

INSTRUCTIONS:

1. In a small bowl, mix together milk and oats and let sit for ten minutes.

2. Place all other ingredients in a blender, with the exception of the chocolate chips, if using. Add the oat mixture and blend again.

3. Stir in the chocolate chips, if using.

4. Pour the batter onto the waffle maker, and make waffles according to the instructions.

5. I recommend letting the waffles cook a bit longer than the timer indicates (I had my waffle iron set at level 4, but left the waffles on for an extra two minutes). I do this with most of my waffle recipes, as I usually make them with less fat, so they don't crisp up quite as fast and therefore need a bit of extra cooking time.

6. Set the waffle aside to cool, and repeat with remaining batter.

7. Serve as is, or top with *Coconut Whipped Cream* and *Chocolate Sauce* (from the *Sweet n Savoury Dips and Dressings* sections).

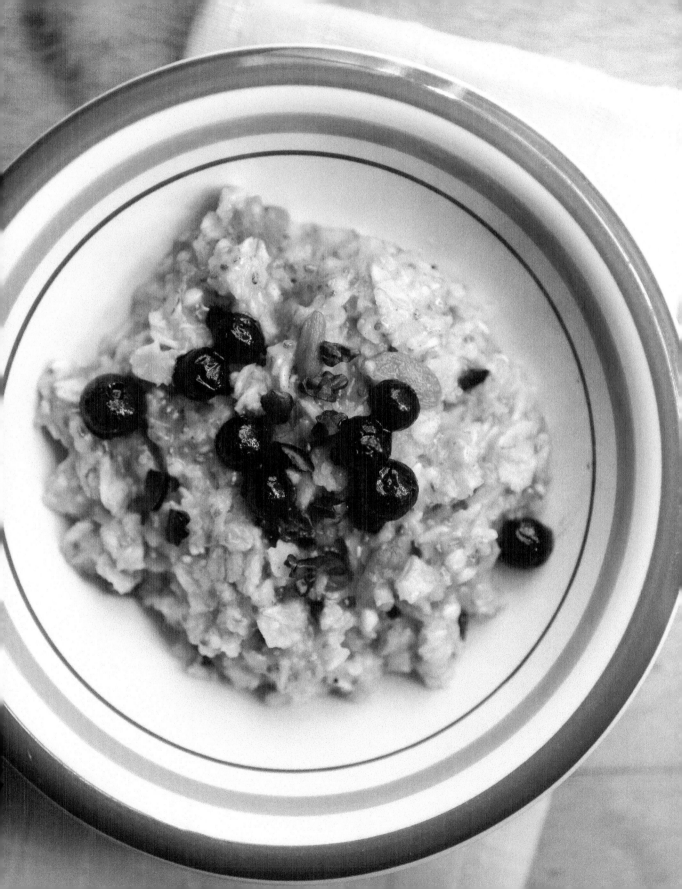

Cacao-Goji Oatmeal

Serves 2

Oats have so many health benefits — for instance, stabilizing blood sugar, lowering cholesterol, reducing high blood pressure, and keeping us regular — but are often viewed as bland. In this recipe, oats get a makeover! Buckwheat, chia seeds, and hemp hearts add texture and goji berries and raw cacao nibs add flavour, as well as a good dose of antioxidants, vitamins, and minerals.

INGREDIENTS:

- 1 cup water
- a pinch of sea salt
- $^1/_2$ cup gluten-free rolled oats
- 2 tablespoons mixture of buckwheat, chia seeds, and hemp hearts
- 2 tablespoons dried goji berries
- 1 tablespoon raw cacao nibs
- 1 teaspoon pure vanilla extract
- 1–2 teaspoons raw honey or real maple syrup, to taste

INSTRUCTIONS:

1. Bring water and salt to a boil.
2. Add the oats, buckwheat, chia seeds, and hemp hearts and stir together.
3. Reduce heat and simmer for 6–8 minutes.
4. Remove from heat and stir in the goji berries, cacao nibs, vanilla, and honey or maple syrup.
5. Serve as is, or top with fresh berries.

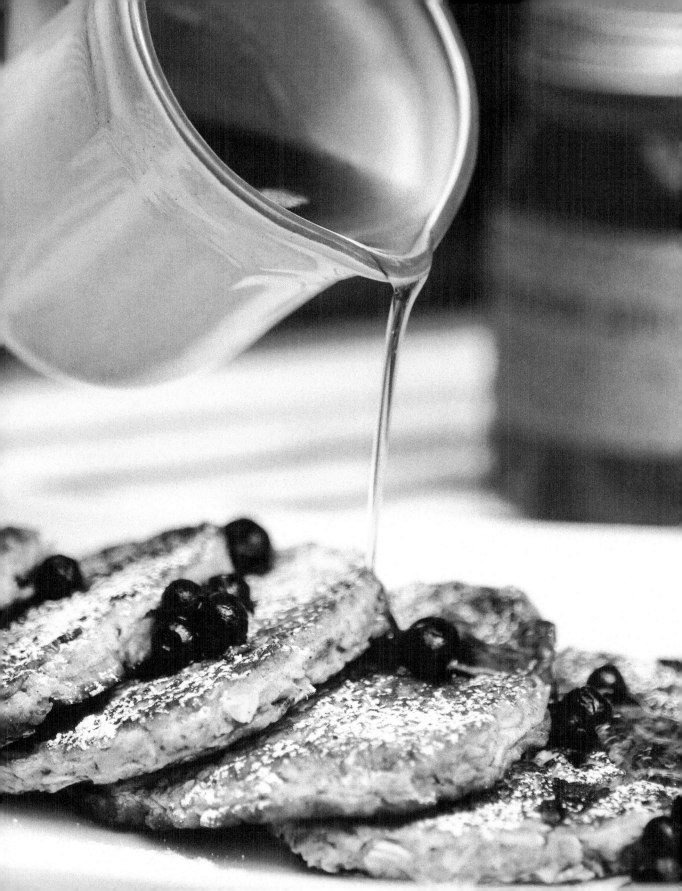

High-Protein Pancakes

Serves 4–6

Talk about a perfectly balanced breakfast! These hearty, sugar-free pancakes will support your fitness and nutrition goals while pleasing your taste buds at the same time. The bananas and raisins add a touch of sweetness that makes them seem more decadent than they really are.

INGREDIENTS:

- 1 cup gluten-free rolled oats
- 1 cup egg whites or 5 large eggs
- 1 tablespoon ground flaxseed
- $1/2$ cup vanilla vegan protein powder
- 1 ripe banana, mashed
- 1 teaspoon ground cinnamon
- $1/4$ cup raisins
- coconut oil, for the pan

INSTRUCTIONS:

1. In a medium-sized bowl, mix together all ingredients, with the exception of the raisins and the coconut oil.

2. Heat a skillet on medium-high heat and add some coconut oil so the pancakes won't stick. Pour in a $1/4$ cup of the batter and then add in a few raisins. Cook the pancake until bubbles appear, then flip the pancake and cook other side for about one more minute.

3. Set the pancake aside to cool, then repeat with the remaining batter.

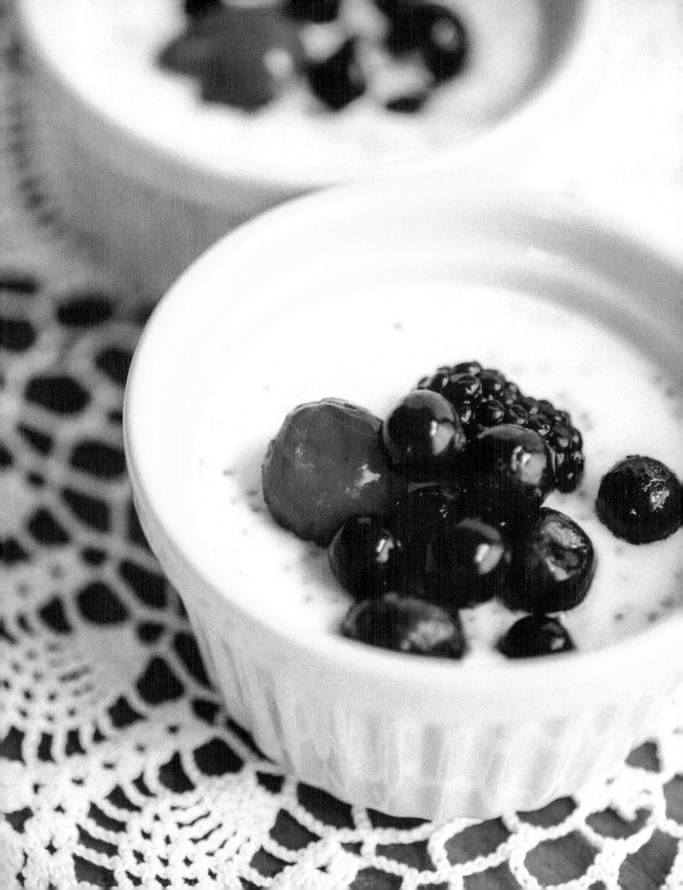

Vanilla-Chia Pudding

Serves 2-3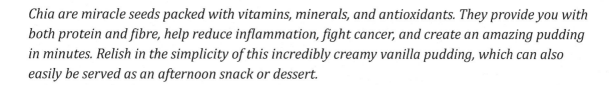

Chia are miracle seeds packed with vitamins, minerals, and antioxidants. They provide you with both protein and fibre, help reduce inflammation, fight cancer, and create an amazing pudding in minutes. Relish in the simplicity of this incredibly creamy vanilla pudding, which can also easily be served as an afternoon snack or dessert.

INGREDIENTS:

- $^3/_4$ cup coconut cream, scooped off the top of a can of chilled, full-fat coconut milk
- $^1/_2$ cup unsweetened almond milk
- 3 tablespoons chia seeds
- 1 tablespoon real maple syrup
- 1 $^1/_2$ teaspoons pure vanilla extract
- 1 cup mixed fresh berries, for topping

INSTRUCTIONS:

1. Mix together the cream, almond milk, chia seeds, maple syrup, and vanilla until well-combined and the mixture starts to thicken.

2. Cover and let chill in the fridge overnight.

3. Remove from fridge, top with fresh berries, and serve.

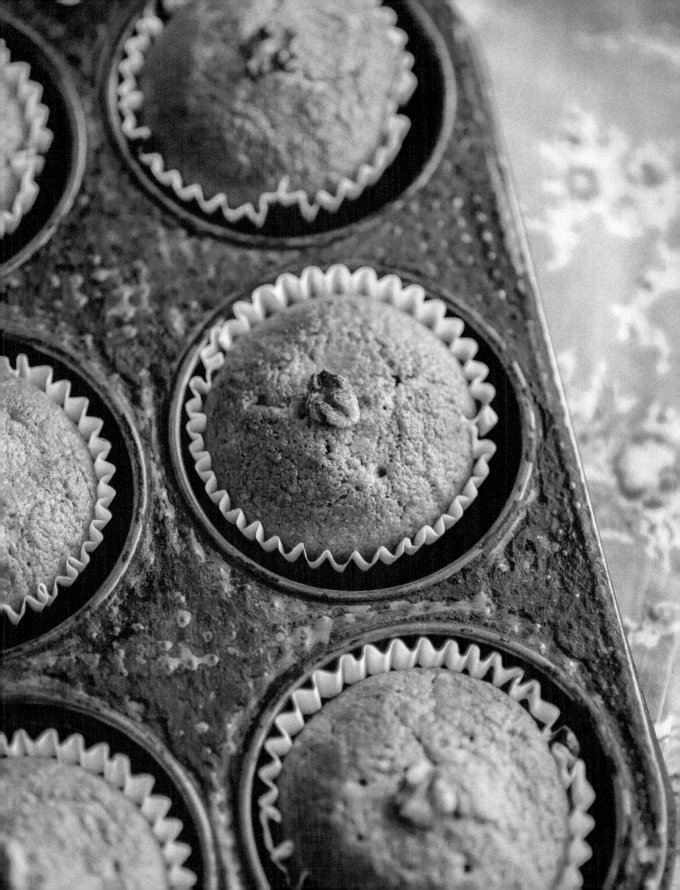

Banana-Nut Muffins

Serves 12

Banana-nut muffins are one of breakfast's greatest pleasures. Wake up in the morning to smell these baking in the oven and be comforted by that fact that they taste as good as they smell, without any of the artery-clogging ingredients found in traditional muffins.

INGREDIENTS:

- $^2/_3$ cup gluten-free oat flour
- $^2/_3$ cup brown rice flour
- $^2/_3$ cup almond flour
- 2 tablespoons chia seeds
- 3 teaspoons baking powder
- $^1/_2$ teaspoon sea salt
- 2 teaspoons ground cinnamon
- $^1/_2$ cup real maple syrup
- 2 large eggs
- 1 cup mashed, ripe bananas
- $^1/_2$ cup unsweetened vanilla almond milk
- 1 tablespoon apple cider vinegar
- 2 teaspoons pure vanilla extract
- $^1/_2$ cup walnut pieces

INSTRUCTIONS:

1. Preheat oven to 400°F.
2. Add the flours, chia seeds, baking powder, salt, and cinnamon, to your food processor and mix until well blended.
3. Add all remaining ingredients, with the exception of the walnuts, and mix until well blended and no chunks remain. Stir in the walnuts by hand.
4. Pour into a muffin tin lined with silicone muffin cups and bake for 22–25 minutes. Remove and let cool on a wire rack.

> **TIP:**
> I love foods that look like the body part that they are good for. For example, walnuts, which are high in omega-3's, are important for good brain function. If you look closely, you will see that walnuts closely resemble a human brain.

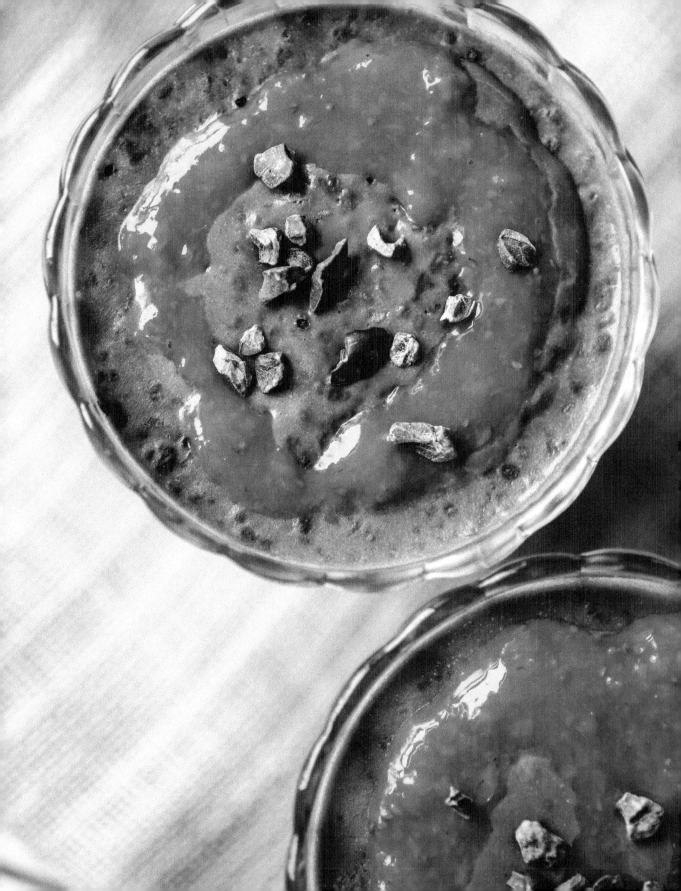

Chocolate-Chia Pudding

Serves 2-3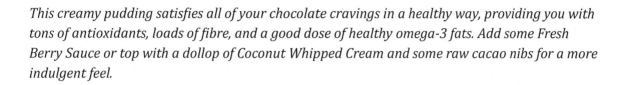

This creamy pudding satisfies all of your chocolate cravings in a healthy way, providing you with tons of antioxidants, loads of fibre, and a good dose of healthy omega-3 fats. Add some Fresh Berry Sauce or top with a dollop of Coconut Whipped Cream and some raw cacao nibs for a more indulgent feel.

INGREDIENTS:

- ¹/₂ cup coconut cream, scooped off the top of a can of chilled, full-fat coconut milk
- ¹/₂ cup unsweetened vanilla almond milk
- 2 tablespoons chia seeds
- 2 tablespoons real maple syrup
- a pinch of sea salt
- 3 tablespoons raw cacao powder
- toppings: *Coconut Whipped Cream* (from the *Sweet n' Savoury Dips and Dressings* section) and raw cacao nibs or fresh berry sauce

INSTRUCTIONS:

1. In a glass container, mix together cream, milk, chia seeds, maple syrup, and sea salt until well combined.
2. Cover and let chill in your fridge overnight.
3. In the morning, remove from the fridge and stir in the raw cacao powder.
4. Top with the *Coconut Whipped Cream* (from the *Sweet n' Savoury Dips and Dressings* section) and a few raw cacao nibs, or some *Fresh Berry Sauce* (from the tip below).

> **TIP:** 🍴
> To make fresh berry sauce, mix together one cup of frozen berries, one tablespoon of maple syrup and a pinch of sea salt in a large pot and bring to a boil. Reduce the heat slightly and continue to cook over medium heat until the mixture thickens. Remove from heat and serve warm, or if you prefer a smooth sauce, blend in the food processor for a few seconds before serving.

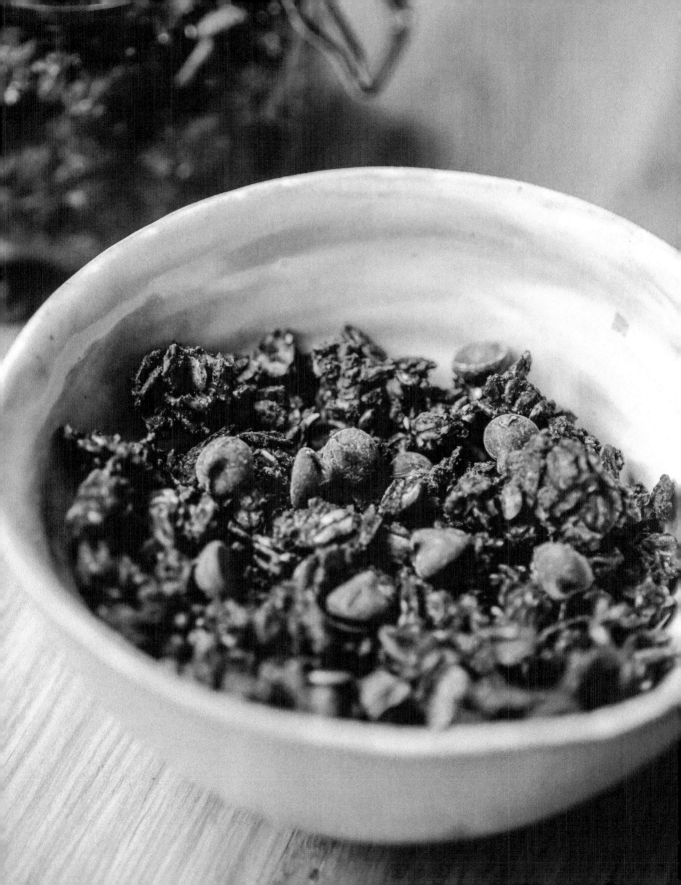

Double-Chocolate Granola

Serves 4-6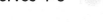

Indulge in your chocolate love affair with this decadent, delightful and delicious granola. Rich in antioxidants and high in fibre and complex carbs, this granola will keep your belly — and brain — happy for hours. Serve with almond milk or yogurt for breakfast or grab a handful as an on-the-go, high-energy snack.

INGREDIENTS:

- 3 cups gluten-free rolled oats
- 1 cup quick-cooking gluten-free oats
- $^1/_3$ cup cocoa powder
- $^1/_2$ cup shredded, unsweetened coconut
- 2 tablespoons flax or chia meal
- 2 tablespoons hemp hearts
- $^1/_2$ teaspoon ground cinnamon
- $^1/_4$ teaspoon sea salt
- $^1/_2$ cup coconut oil
- $^1/_3$ cup dairy-free chocolate chips
- $^1/_4$ cup real maple syrup
- 1 $^1/_2$ teaspoons pure vanilla extract
- $^1/_2$ cup dairy-free chocolate chips (again)

INSTRUCTIONS:

1. Preheat oven to 325°F.
2. In a large bowl, mix together both types of oats, cocoa powder, coconut, flax or chia meal, hemp hearts, cinnamon, and sea salt. Set aside.
3. In a small pot, heat coconut oil and chocolate chips (the $^1/_3$ cup) just until melted.
4. Remove from heat and stir in the maple syrup and vanilla.
5. Pour the chocolate mixture over the oat mixture and stir together until completely coated.
6. Spread evenly onto a parchment-paper-lined cookie sheet.
7. Bake for 45 minutes, making sure to stir every 15 minutes because the outside edges tend to brown faster.
8. Remove from oven and immediately mix in the remaining chocolate chips.
9. Let cool completely before storing in an air-tight, glass container.

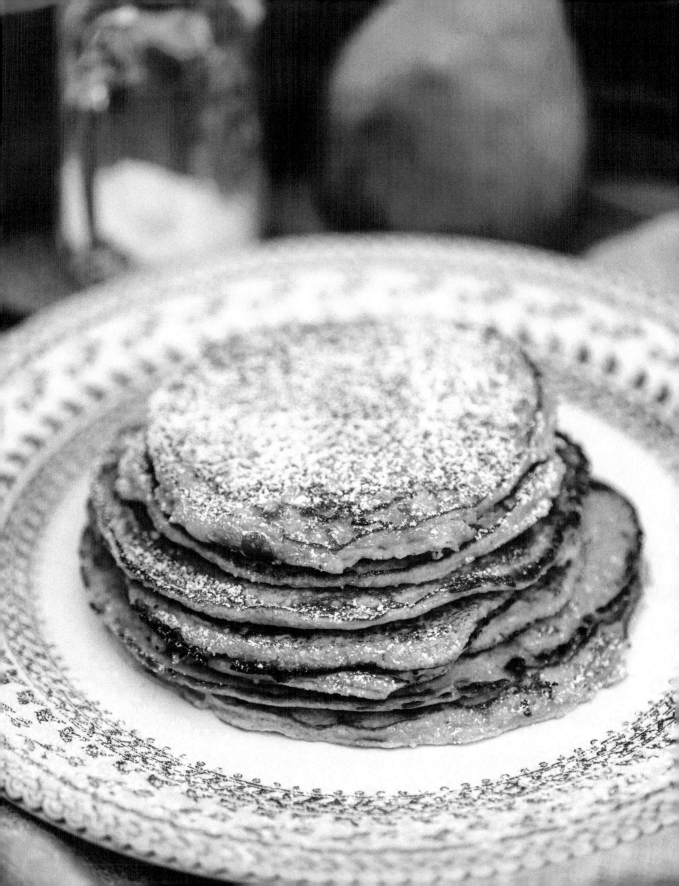

Peanut-Butter Pumpkin Pancakes

Serves 4–6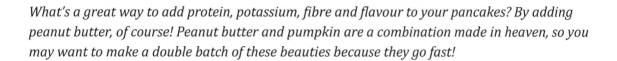

What's a great way to add protein, potassium, fibre and flavour to your pancakes? By adding peanut butter, of course! Peanut butter and pumpkin are a combination made in heaven, so you may want to make a double batch of these beauties because they go fast!

INGREDIENTS:

- 1 cup gluten-free rolled oats
- 2 tablespoons natural peanut butter
- 2 tablespoons raw honey
- 2 tablespoons pumpkin purée
- 1 $1/2$ teaspoons pure vanilla extract
- 2 large eggs
- $1/2$ teaspoon baking powder
- $1/2$ teaspoon ground cinnamon
- $1/2$ cup unsweetened almond milk or coconut milk (from a carton)
- coconut oil, for the pan

INSTRUCTIONS:

1. Blend together all ingredients with the exception of the coconut oil in a blender or food processor.
2. Heat a bit of coconut oil in a frying pan over medium heat.
3. Pour about $1/2$ cup of batter into the pan and cook until the edges start to brown and bubbles start to form.
4. Flip the pancake and cook until cooked through.
5. Repeat with remaining batter.
6. Serve warm.

> **TIP:**
> Orange and yellow vegetables like pumpkins, sweet potatoes, squash, and carrots are high in beta-carotene, which is a potent antioxidant that protects our cells from free radical damage and aging. It's especially good for eye and skin health.

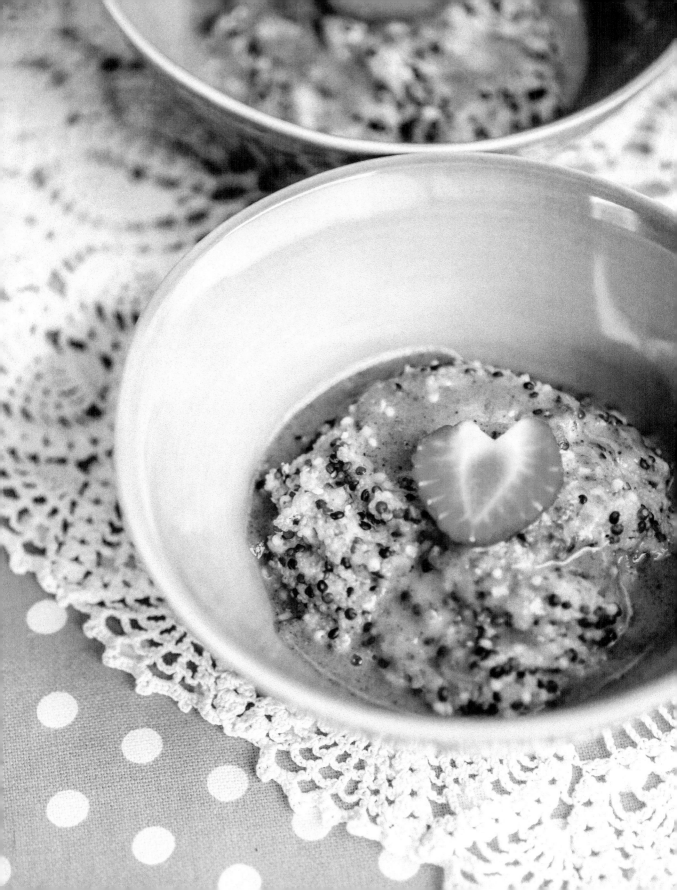

Four-Grain Porridge

Serves 2

Why settle for a single grain when you can benefit from four ancient grains instead? A great way to switch up an oatmeal rut, this comforting porridge gets an upgrade with a creamy almond topping which will have you have coming back for seconds.

INGREDIENTS:

Topping ingredients:

- 2 tablespoons almond butter
- ¹/₄ cup unsweetened almond milk
- 2 tablespoons raw honey
- a pinch of sea salt

Porridge ingredients:

- 2 tablespoons millet
- 2 tablespoons quinoa
- 2 tablespoons amaranth
- 1 cup unsweetened vanilla almond milk
- ¹/₂ cup water
- 2 tablespoons gluten-free steel cut oats
- 2 tablespoons gluten-free rolled oats
- a pinch of sea salt
- add-ins of choice: strawberries, blackberries, pomegranate, pistachios, or hemp hearts

INSTRUCTIONS:

1. To make topping, in a small pot over medium heat, mix together almond butter, almond milk, honey, and sea salt, just until combined. Remove from heat and set aside.

2. To make porridge, place millet, quinoa, and amaranth in a fine mesh strainer, and rinse well.

3. Add almond milk, water, all four grains, and sea salt to a medium-sized pot, and bring to a boil over medium-high heat, stirring regularly so the milk doesn't burn.

4. Reduce heat, cover and simmer for 15 minutes. Remove from heat and let sit for five more minutes, uncovered.

5. Spoon porridge into serving bowls and drizzle with the desired amount of the almond topping and add-ins of choice.

6. Store remaining topping in the fridge in an air-tight, glass container for up to a week.

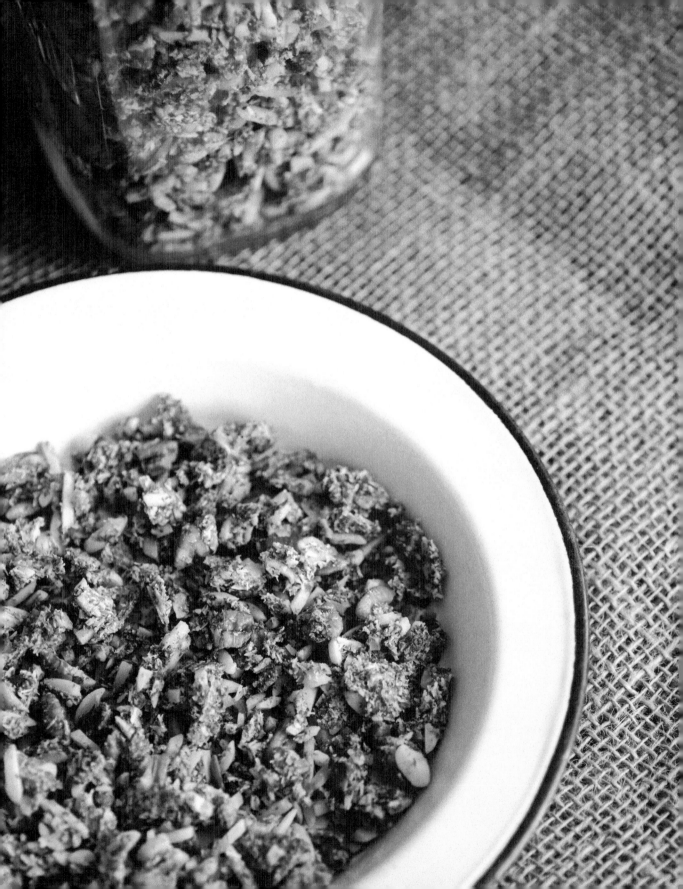

Orange Maple-Nut Granola

Serves 10–12

You will be excited to wake up to this completely grain-free granola, which smells just divine. The orange zest really intensifies the flavour, and when combined with the roasted almonds, you have a match made in heaven.

INGREDIENTS:

- 2 cups slivered almonds
- 1 cup pecans, chopped
- $^1/_2$ cup chia seeds, ground
- 1 cup shredded, unsweetened coconut
- $^1/_2$ cup almond meal
- $^1/_2$ cup freshly-squeezed orange juice
- 2 tablespoons orange zest
- 5 tablespoons real maple syrup
- 2 tablespoons coconut oil
- $^1/_4$ cup unsweetened applesauce

INSTRUCTIONS:

1. Preheat oven to 325°F.
2. Mix together nuts, chia, coconut, and almond meal in a large bowl, and set aside.
3. In a small saucepan over medium heat, mix together orange juice, zest, maple syrup, coconut oil, and applesauce until everything has melted together and is well combined.
4. Pour the liquid ingredients over the dry seeds and nuts and mix together well.
5. Pour granola onto a deep baking sheet lined with parchment paper, and spread it out evenly.
6. Bake for 40–50 minutes or until granola is golden brown, making sure to stir every 15 minutes because the outside edges tend to brown faster.
7. Allow to cool completely before storing in an air-tight, glass container.

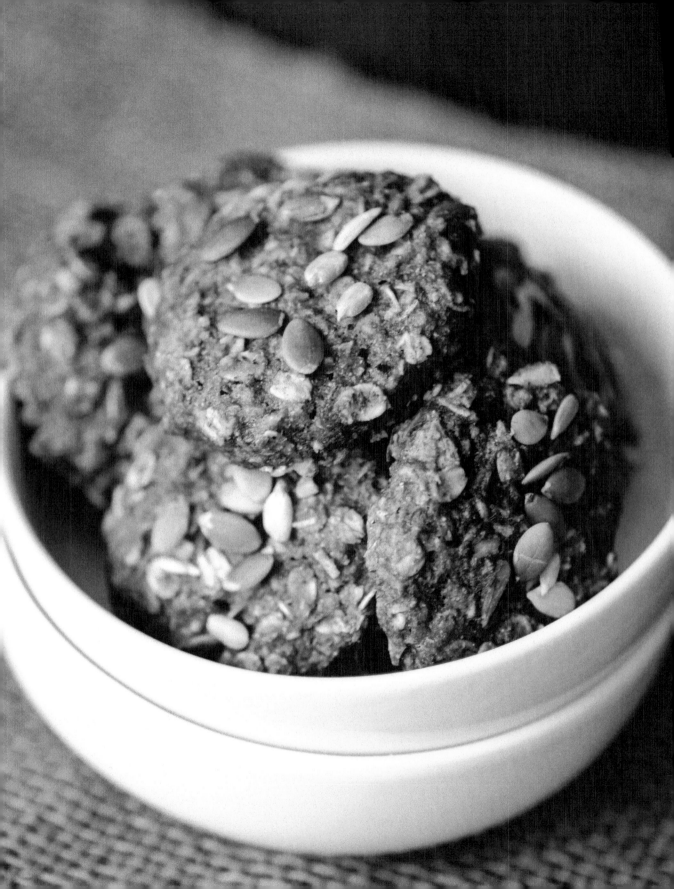

Grab n' Go Breakfast Cookies

Serves 8-10

These hearty, chewy cookies are healthy enough to be eaten any time of day and are great for those on the go. Full of whole grains, healthy fats, fibre, and protein, and sweetened mainly with bananas and applesauce, these cookies really do a body good.

INGREDIENTS:

- 2 tablespoons ground chia seeds
- $^1/_2$ cup warm water
- 1 $^1/_2$ cups gluten-free rolled oats
- $^3/_4$ cup buckwheat flour
- 1 teaspoon ground cinnamon
- $^1/_2$ teaspoon baking soda
- $^1/_2$ teaspoon sea salt
- 2 ripe bananas, peeled and chopped
- $^1/_3$ cup unsweetened applesauce
- $^1/_4$ cup real maple syrup
- $^1/_4$ cup natural unsweetened sunflower-seed butter
- $^1/_2$ cup each raisins and unsweetened shredded coconut
- $^1/_4$ cup each pecans, sunflower, and pumpkin seeds

INSTRUCTIONS:

1. Preheat oven to 350°F.

2. In a small bowl, mix chia seeds with warm water, stir, and let sit for 5 minutes.

3. In a large bowl mix together oats, buckwheat, cinnamon, baking soda, and salt and set aside.

4. In a food processor, mix together bananas, applesauce, maple syrup, sunflower-seed butter, and chia mixture.

5. Add wet ingredients to dry ingredients and mix by hand. Add in raisins, coconut, nuts, and seeds, and stir to incorporate.

6. Line a baking sheet with parchment paper and form dough into large palm-sized cookies, flattening each cookie slightly with the back of a fork.

7. Place the cookies in oven and bake for 15 minutes.

8. Remove and let cool on a wire rack.

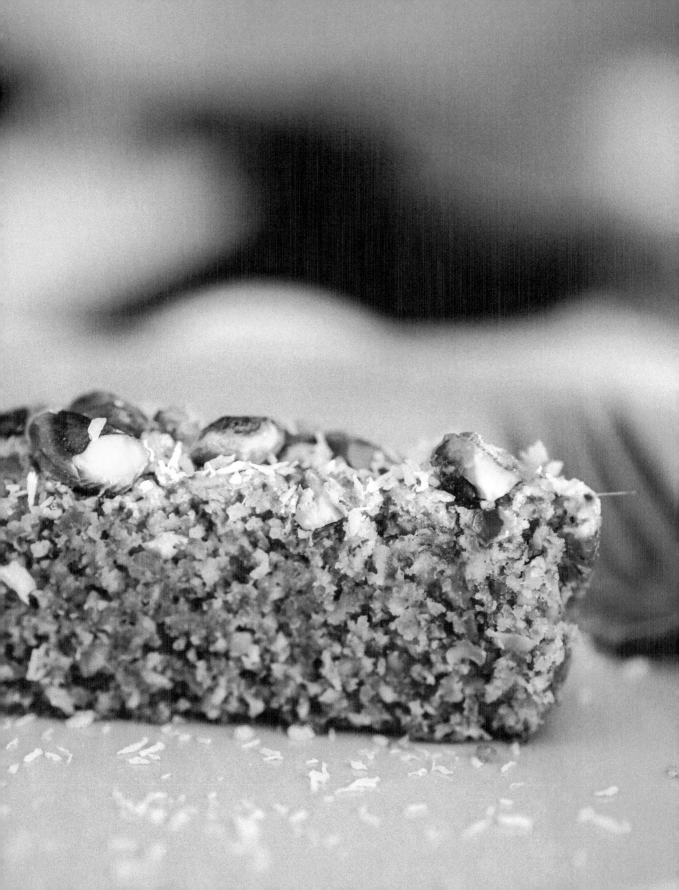

Apricot Pistachio Loaf

Serves 8-10

These nutty loaves are so moist and addictive that it's hard not to eat them all in one sitting. The olive oil flavour pairs incredibly well with the sweetness of the apricots and the saltiness of the pistachios, making this loaf taste absolutely divine.

INGREDIENTS:

- 3 cups gluten-free rolled oats
- 1 cup pistachios, roasted and salted
- $^3/_4$ cup dried apricots
- $^1/_2$ cup extra-virgin olive oil
- $^1/_2$ cup pitted Medjool dates
- $^1/_2$ cup pumpkin seeds
- $^1/_2$ cup shredded, unsweetened coconut
- $^3/_4$ cup real maple syrup
- 1 teaspoon sea salt
- $^1/_2$ teaspoon ground cinnamon

INSTRUCTIONS:

1. Preheat oven to 350°F.
2. Mix all ingredients together in a food processor until the dough sticks together but some texture remains.
3. Press firmly into a parchment-paper-lined baking pan, making sure to smooth out the top with either a rolling pin or a by pressing down with a cutting board.
4. Bake for 25–30 minutes or until the edges are lightly browned.
5. Remove from the oven and allow to cool before cutting into squares or bars.

NOTE:

This recipe was adapted from the Olive Oil Granola with Dried Apricots and Pistachios recipe by Melissa Clark featured in the New York Times online on July 10, 2009 (http://www.melissaclark.net).[43]

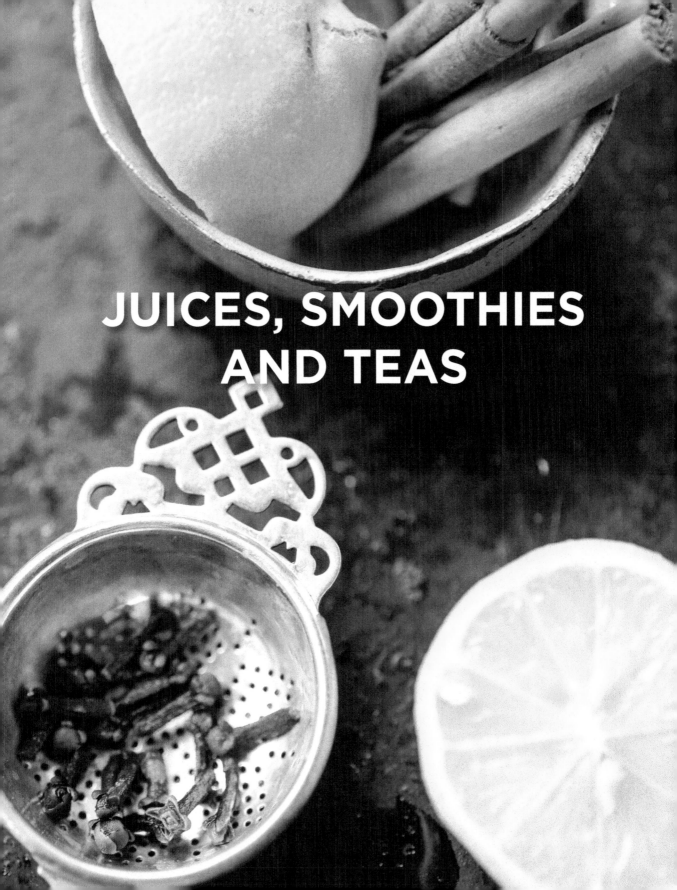

JUICES, SMOOTHIES AND TEAS

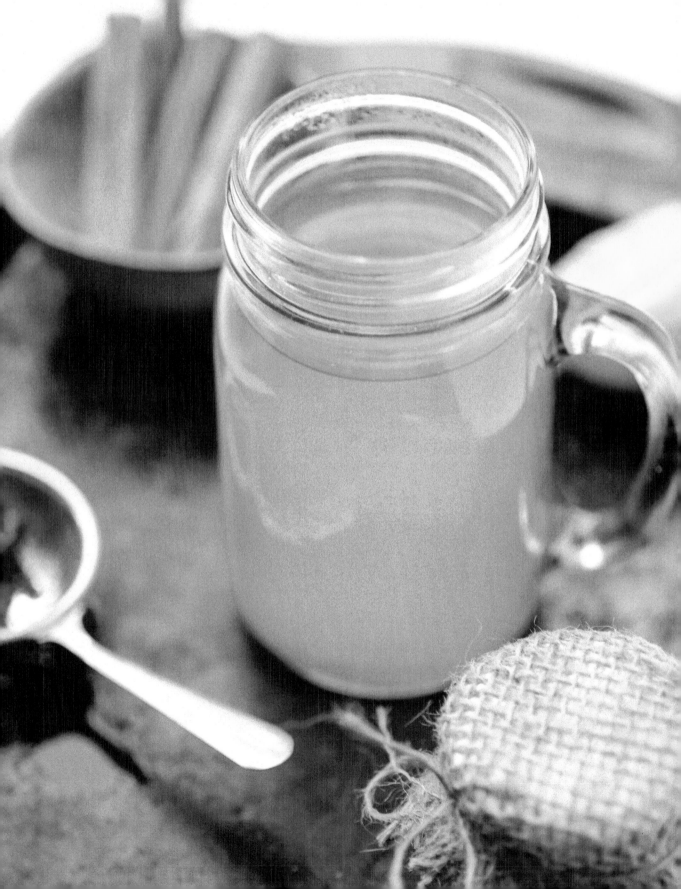

Flu-Fighting Tea

Serves 2

There is nothing like warm tea to help boost your spirits when you are feeling under the weather. This tea is extra special because it is made with naturally potent spices which will help boost your immune system and ward off colds and flus. Both sweet, spicy, and wonderfully aromatic, this tea will delight all of your senses.

INGREDIENTS:

- 3 cups water
- 1 cinnamon stick
- $^1/_2$ inch slice of fresh ginger
- 5–6 whole cloves
- 5–6 cardamom pods
- a pinch of cayenne
- $^1/_2$ teaspoon ground turmeric
- $^1/_2$ lemon, juiced
- 1 tablespoon raw honey

INSTRUCTIONS:

1. Add all ingredients, with the exception of the lemon and honey, to a small pot and bring to a boil. Turn down the heat and simmer for 15 minutes.

2. Remove from heat. Strain, and stir in the honey and lemon juice.

3. Now sit back, relax, and enjoy sipping your way back to good health!

> **NOTE:**
> Inspired by Nutritionista Meghan Telpner's Yogi Tea. See the original recipe here - http://www.meghantelpner.com/blog/warm-tea-on-a-cold-night[44.]

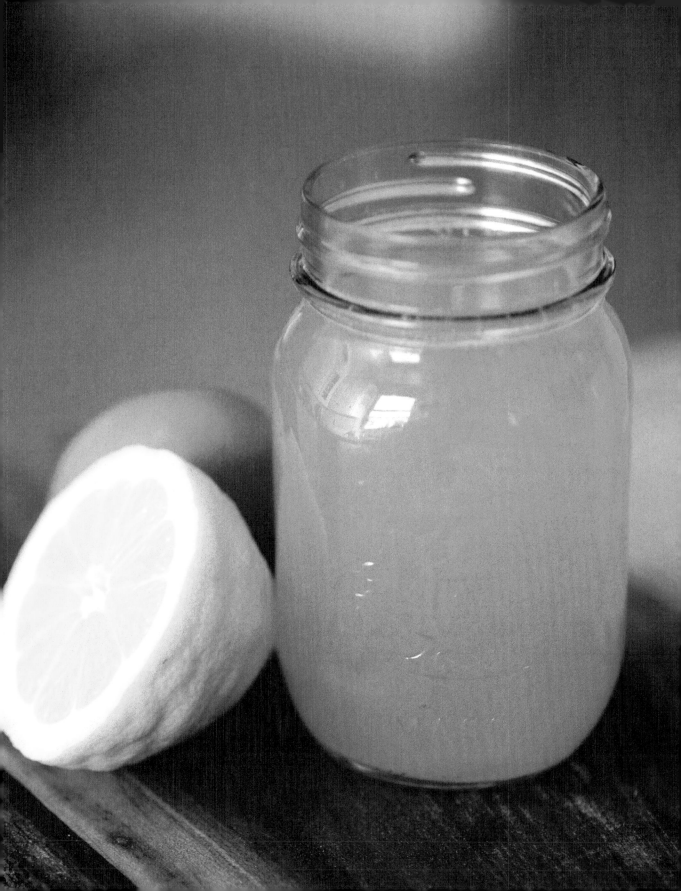

Lemon Aid Energy Drink

Serves 1-2

Kids and adults alike will love the taste of this simple electrolyte-rich drink that has none of the artificial colours or flavours that are present in most commercial energy drinks. Drink this to recover and rehydrate after a hot day or a long workout.

INGREDIENTS:

- 2 cups water
- 1 Rooibos tea bag
- $^1/_8$ cup freshly-squeezed lemon juice
- $^1/_8$ cup freshly-squeezed lime juice
- 2 tablespoons raw honey
- a pinch of sea salt

INSTRUCTIONS:

1. Bring water to a boil in a small saucepan.
2. Remove from heat, add the Rooibos tea bag, and let steep for 10–15 minutes.
3. Remove the tea bag, add the freshly-squeezed juices, honey and sea salt, and stir until the honey dissolves.
4. Let cool and then transfer to the fridge to chill for at least two hours.
5. This drink can be diluted with some additional water if preferred.

> **TIP:** 🍴
> This drink is also a fantastic choice when recovering from flus and colds and helping kids rehydrate when they are sick. It can be served warm as well as cold.

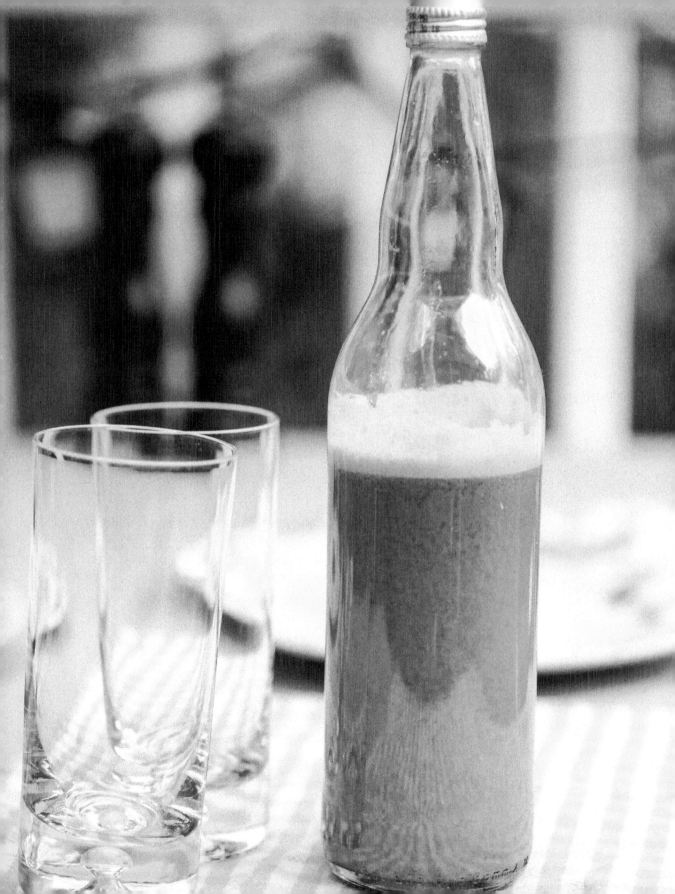

Green Living Juice

Serves 1

This super green juice will infuse your cells with such a massive dose of nutrients that they will be buzzing with energy for the rest of the day. Super hydrating and super rich in chlorophyll, this juice will make you glow from the inside out.

INGREDIENTS:

- 5 small handfuls of kale or spinach
- 1 cucumber
- 3 stalks celery
- 2 green apples, seeded and halved
- 1 lemon, peeled
- 1 inch piece of peeled, fresh ginger

INSTRUCTIONS:

1. Run all ingredients through a juicer.
2. Strain through a nut-milk bag if you don't like pulp.
3. Enjoy immediately.

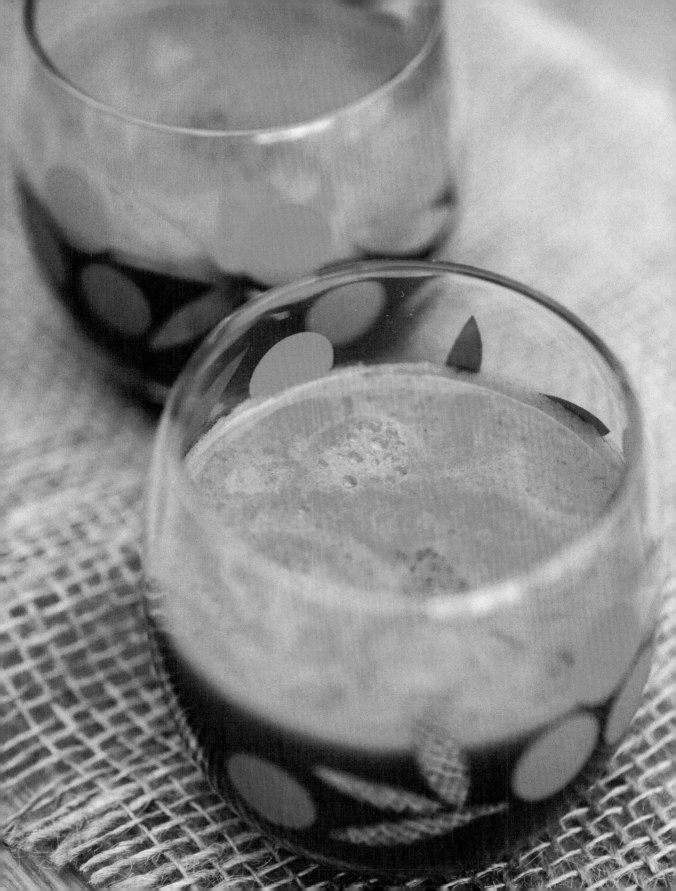

Liver-Cleanse Juice

Serves 1

Whose liver couldn't use a helping hand once in a while? Detoxifying your body is hard work, and this liver-cleanse juice will provide your body with the support it needs to make the job a little easier.

INGREDIENTS:

- 1 beet, halved
- 2 carrots
- 1 apple, cored and halved
- 2 stalks celery
- 2 cups romaine lettuce
- a handful of fresh parsley
- $^1/_2$ lemon, peeled

INSTRUCTIONS:

1. Run all ingredients through a juicer.
2. Strain through a nut-milk bag if you don't like pulp.
3. Enjoy immediately.

> **TIP:**
> Beet juice looks a lot like blood, and for good reason. Beets are high in antioxidants and nitrates, which are great for dilating blood vessels and lowering blood pressure. Beets aren't the only part of the plant that is good for you either! The leafy green tops of the beets are highly nutritious and taste great. They are also high in iron, protein, zinc, fiber, magnesium, and potassium. Just sauté them in a little coconut oil and sprinkle them with sea salt before serving.

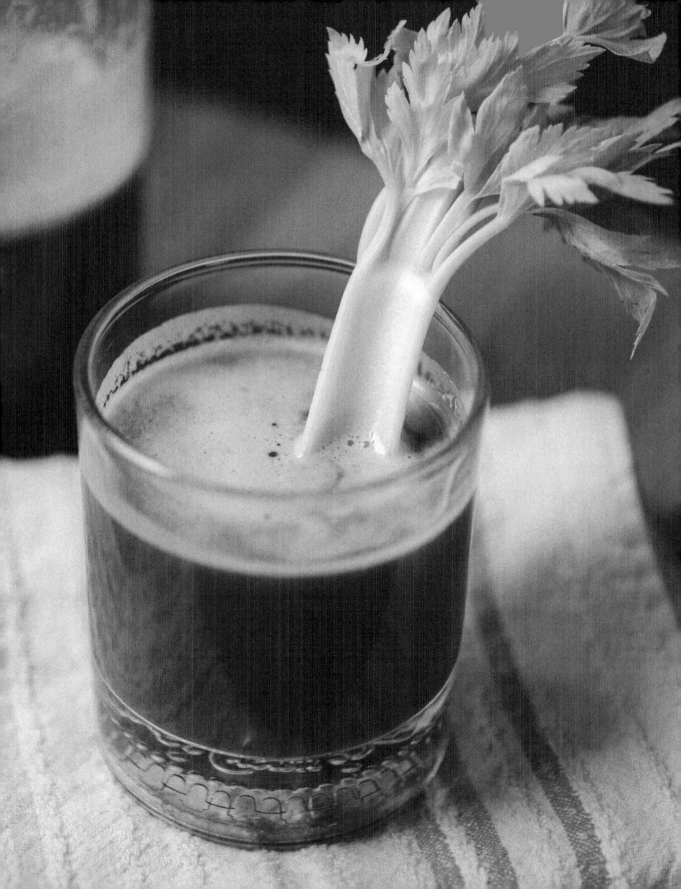

My Morning Greens

Serves 1

I love drinking this juice first thing in the morning because it tastes amazing and provides me with at least half of my fruit and veggie servings for the day. Plus, it's wonderfully detoxifying and incredibly hydrating, so it's like getting a facial from the inside out!

INGREDIENTS:

- 2 apples, cored and halved
- 1 English cucumber
- 3 cups kale
- 2 stalks celery
- a handful fresh parsley
- $^1/_2$ lemon, peeled
- $^1/_2$ inch piece of peeled, fresh ginger

INSTRUCTIONS:

1. Run all ingredients through a juicer.
2. Strain through a nut-milk bag if you don't like pulp.
3. Enjoy immediately.

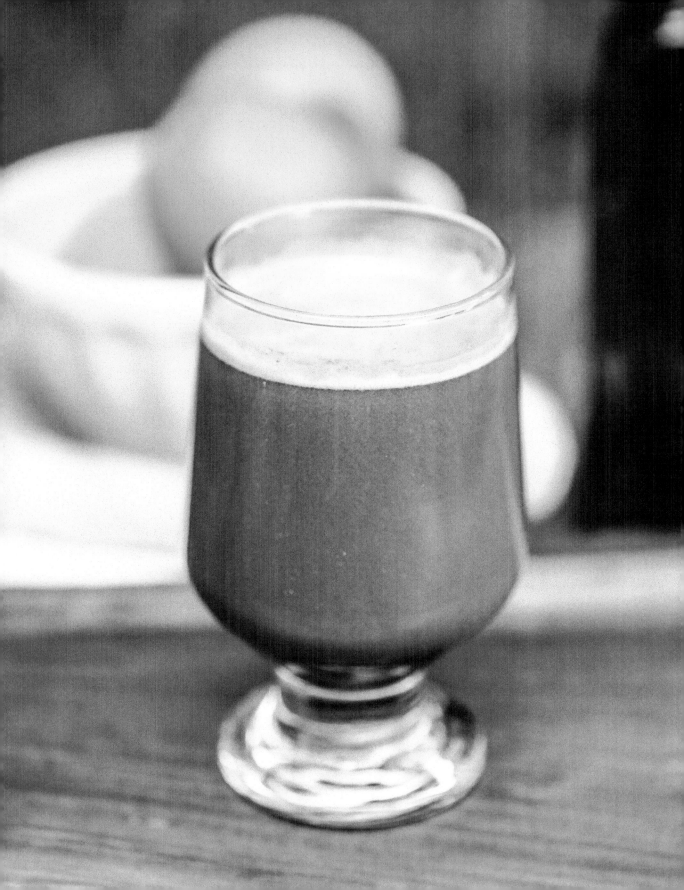

Green Ginger Juice

Serves 1

This juice will give you the kick you need to get moving in the morning (or anytime!). Detoxifying parsley and anti-inflammatory ginger add a zing to this sweet green elixir which will make you feel like you just left the spa!

INGREDIENTS:

- $1/2$ green apple
- $1/2$ pear
- 1–2 leaves Swiss chard or romaine lettuce
- $1/2$–1 cup fresh parsley
- 1 large or 2 small broccoli stalks
- 2 stalks celery
- $1/2$ cucumber
- $1/2$ inch piece of peeled, fresh ginger
- $1/2$ lemon, peeled

INSTRUCTIONS:

1. Run all ingredients through a juicer.
2. Strain through a nut-milk bag if you don't like pulp.
3. Enjoy immediately.

> **TIP:** 🍴
> Parsley is an incredibly powerful herb – it is rich in vitamins A, C, K, and B-12, and is fantastic for boosting the immune system, assisting with digestion (which is why you often see it on your plate as a garnish), and preventing cancer.

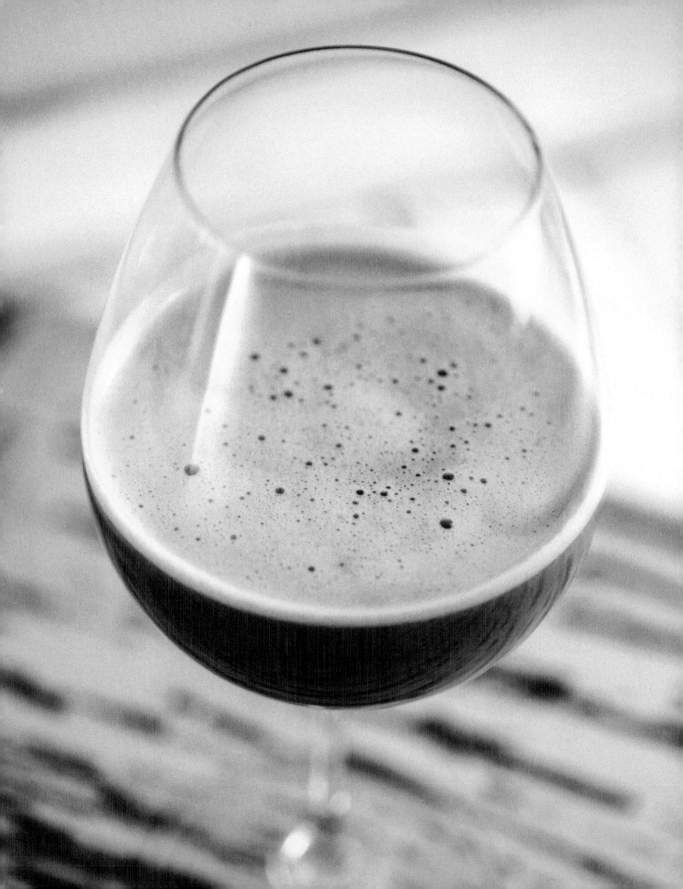

Green Apple Juice

Serves 1

Apple juice gets a makeover with the addition of phytonutrient-packed veggies. The lemon and ginger add a depth of flavour that makes this juice just a bit more grown-up. Drink this detoxifying elixir out of a wine glass before dinner for an extra dose of health-promoting nutrients!

INGREDIENTS:

- 1 apple, cored and halved
- 2 broccoli stalks
- 2 Lebanese cucumbers (or ½ regular cucumber)
- 3 stalks celery
- 1 cup packed baby spinach
- $^1/_2$ lemon, peeled
- $^1/_4$–$^1/_2$ inch piece of peeled, fresh ginger

INSTRUCTIONS:

1. Run all ingredients through a juicer.
2. Strain through a nut-milk bag if you don't like pulp.
3. Enjoy immediately.

TIP:

Nut milk bags, also known as nut sacks (yes, you are permitted to laugh), are nylon bags which are ideal for minimizing sediment when juicing or making homemade nut milks. Nut sacks can be found online at: http://www.trulyorganicfoods.com/nut-milk-bags.php

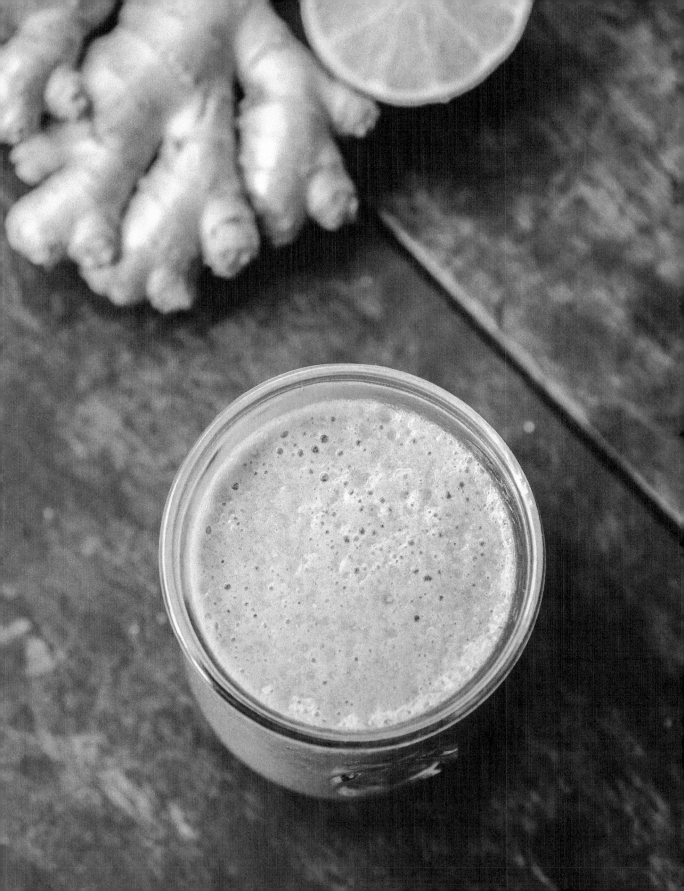

Pineapple-Mint Smoothie

Serves 1

I love drinking this pineapple-mint smoothie on a hot summer afternoon or after a workout. The banana provides electrolytes, the pineapple is great for energizing tired muscles and fighting inflammation, and the mint is wonderful for soothing the digestive system and fighting fatigue.

INGREDIENTS:

- 2 cups frozen pineapple
- $1/2$ frozen, ripe banana, chopped
- 1 cup kale
- 6 mint leaves
- juice of $1/2$ lime
- 1 cup water
- optional: $1/2$ inch piece of peeled, fresh ginger

INSTRUCTIONS:

1. Add all ingredients to a high-powered blender in the order listed and blend until smooth.
2. Serve immediately.

> **TIP:**
>
> If you are a smoothie lover like me, you will always need frozen bananas on hand. To make sure I never run out I am constantly on the lookout for bundles of ripe bananas (sometimes you can find them on the day-old rack and save yourself some money). I bring them home, peel them, and freeze them whole in large ziplock bags. When I need one for a smoothie, I simply take one out of the freezer, chop it into pieces, and use it as needed.

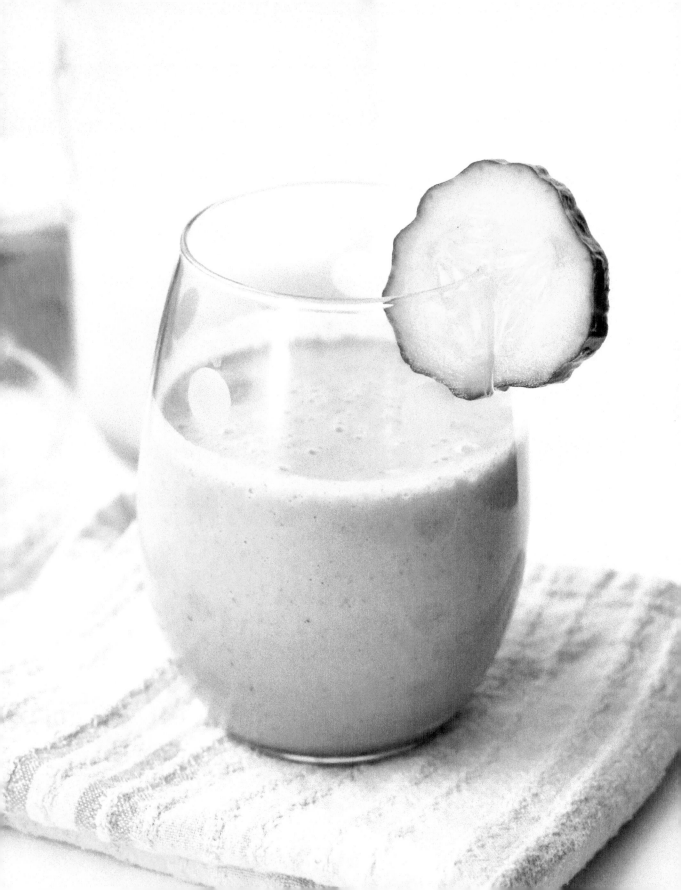

Strawberry-Cucumber Smoothie

Serves 1

Get glowing skin with this simple five-ingredient smoothie. The strawberries and cucumbers are incredibly alkalizing and hydrating, the raw honey is great for soothing the skin, and the lime is rich in antioxidants and vitamin C, which help prevent aging. Now, go get your glow on!

INGREDIENTS:

- 2 cups frozen, whole strawberries
- 1 cup unsweetened almond or coconut milk
- 2 small Lebanese cucumbers or $1/2$ regular cucumber, chopped
- 1 tablespoon raw honey
- juice of $1/2$ lime

INSTRUCTIONS:

1. Add all ingredients to a high-powered blender in the order listed and blend until smooth.
2. Serve immediately.

> **TIP:**
> To make this smoothie a complete meal, add in a $1/2$ scoop of unflavoured vegan protein powder, a tablespoon of chia seeds, $1/2$ cup of almond or coconut milk, and a handful of ice cubes.

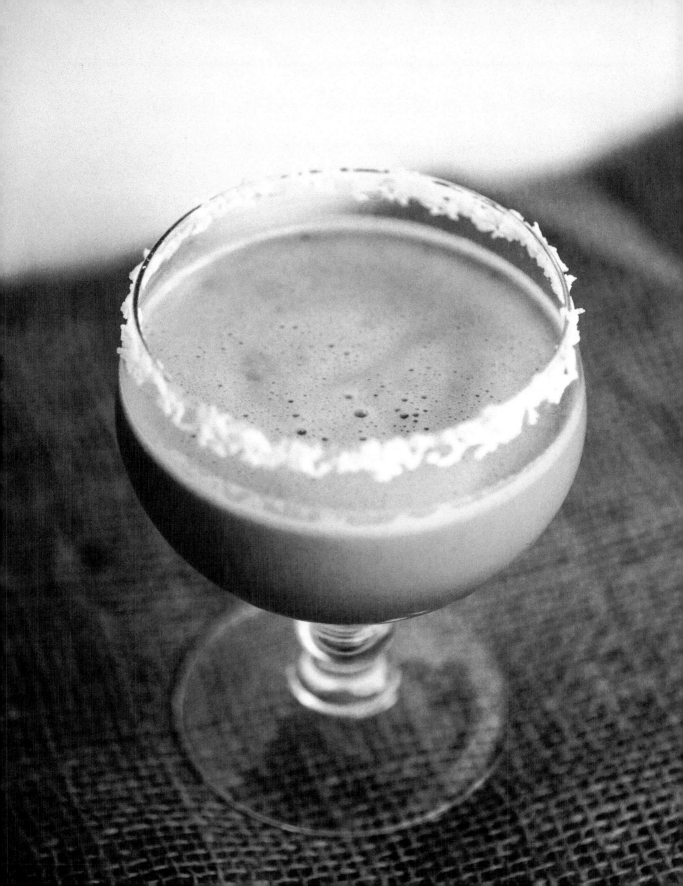

Green Goddess Smoothie

Serves 1

This smoothie is a perfect way to pack greens, fibre, protein and antioxidants into your diet in one shot. Plus, you will feel super trendy walking around sipping your green drink through a glass straw.

INGREDIENTS:

- 1 cup nut or seed milk
- juice of $^1/_2$ lemon
- 1 frozen, ripe banana, chopped
- 2 handfuls of baby spinach
- 1 scoop (about $^1/_4$ cup) vanilla vegan protein powder
- 1 tsp raw honey (optional, if you want to increase the sweetness)
- $^1/_2$ cup ice

INSTRUCTIONS:

1. Add all ingredients to a high-powered blender in the order listed and blend until smooth.
2. Serve immediately.

TIP:
I love drinking smoothies out of glass straws and mason jars. Why? Because glass is non-toxic and re-usable and because it makes me feel super fancy, which is of course, equally important. My favourite straws can be found here: http://www.glassdharma.com

Maqui Pomegranate Smoothie

Serves 2

Kids are going to love this gorgeous, deep purple smoothie because it tastes just like soft-serve ice cream and parents are going to love it because it's incredibly nutritious. High in electrolytes, antioxidants, fibre, vitamin C, vitamin K, and super hydrating, this smoothie makes a great post-workout drink!

INGREDIENTS:

- 2 frozen, ripe bananas, chopped
- 1 pomegranate, seeds and juice
- 2 cups almond milk
- 1 tablespoon maqui berry powder
- 1 tablespoon chia seeds
- 1 teaspoon pure vanilla extract
- 1 tablespoon freshly-squeezed lemon juice

INSTRUCTIONS:

1. Add all ingredients to a high-powered blender in the order listed and blend until smooth.
2. Enjoy immediately.

TIP:

The purple Chilean maqui berry contains the highest antioxidant value of any known superfruit. You can buy it as a freeze-dried powder in health food stores.

Pumpkin Spice Smoothie

Serves 1–2

This delicious, fall-flavoured smoothie tastes just like pumpkin pie! High in antioxidants, vitamin A, zinc, potassium, and fibre, this drink will keep your immune system strong and help you fight off seasonal colds and flus.

INGREDIENTS:

- 1 frozen, ripe banana, chopped
- $^1/_2$ cup pumpkin puree
- $^1/_2$ cup full-fat coconut milk
- $^1/_2$ cup of nut or seed milk
- 1 tablespoon real maple syrup
- 2 Medjool dates, pitted
- 1 teaspoon pure vanilla extract
- 1 teaspoon ground cinnamon
- $^1/_2$–1 inch piece of fresh ginger, peeled
- a pinch–$^1/_8$ teaspoon ground cloves
- 10 ice cubes
- optional toppings: 1–2 tablespoons of *Coconut Whipped Cream* and a bit of grated 70% dark chocolate or a pinch of cinnamon

INSTRUCTIONS:

1. Add all smoothie ingredients to a high-powered blender in the order listed and blend until smooth.
2. Pour the smoothie into a glass mason jar and drink as is, or add optional toppings.
3. If desired, scoop a dollop of *Coconut Whipped Cream* (from the *Sweet n' Savoury Dips and Dressings* section) onto your smoothie and top with grated chocolate or a pinch of cinnamon.

NOTE:

Inspired by my good friend, author, and meditation teacher, Luc Blanchard.

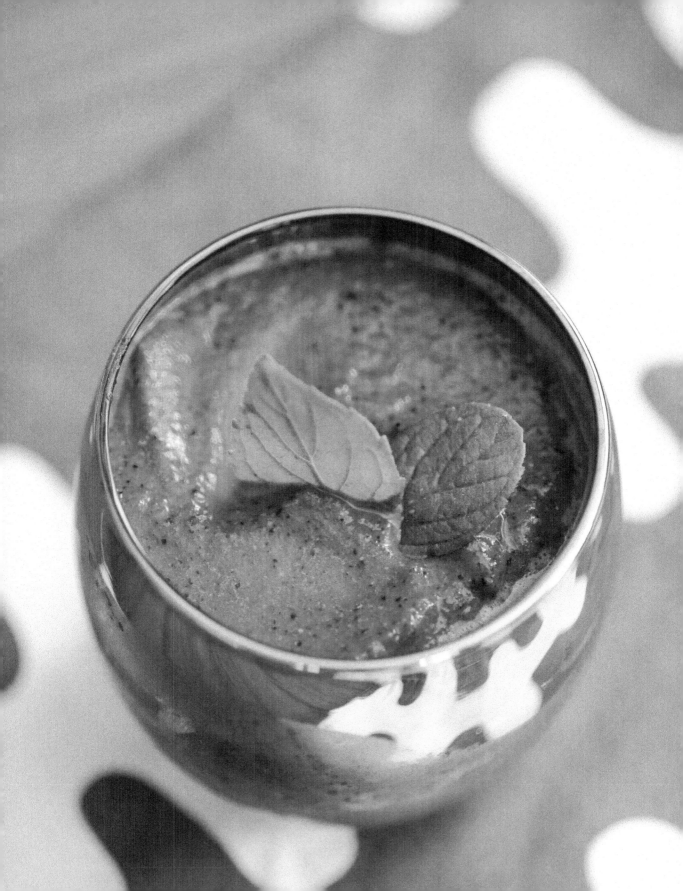

Blueberry-Pineapple Smoothie

Serves 1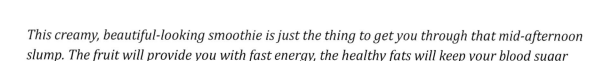

This creamy, beautiful-looking smoothie is just the thing to get you through that mid-afternoon slump. The fruit will provide you with fast energy, the healthy fats will keep your blood sugar balanced, and the fibre will help keep you full.

INGREDIENTS:

- ¹/₄ cup frozen peaches
- ³/₄ cup frozen blueberries
- ¹/₂ cup frozen pineapple
- 1 frozen, ripe banana, chopped
- 1 cup nut or seed milk
- ¹/₂ tablespoon tahini

INSTRUCTIONS:

1. Add all ingredients to a high-powered blender in the order listed and blend until smooth.
2. Serve immediately.

> **TIP:**
> Tahini is also known as sesame seed butter. It's one of the best vegan sources of calcium, is high in protein, and rich in minerals zinc, selenium, iron and copper. Plus, it makes smoothies and sauces super creamy. You may recognize it from its well-known appearance in the popular film *Hummus*.

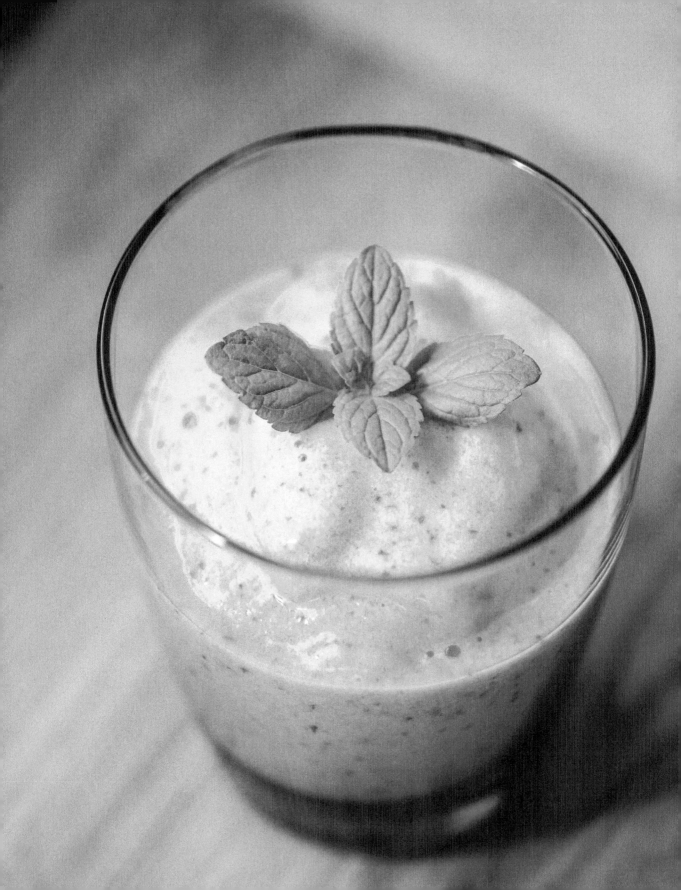

Strawberry Fields Smoothie

Serves 1-2

This healthy version of a strawberry milkshake will bring back memories of your childhood. Luckily, it has less than a quarter of the calories and none of the artificial flavours or colours found in traditional fast-food milkshakes, so you won't feel guilty drinking it.

INGREDIENTS:

- 1 cup frozen strawberries
- 1 frozen, ripe banana, chopped
- $^2/_3$ cup apple juice

INSTRUCTIONS:

1. Add all ingredients to a high-powered blender in the order listed and blend until smooth.
2. Serve immediately.

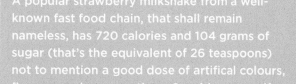

TIP:

A popular strawberry milkshake from a well-known fast food chain, that shall remain nameless, has 720 calories and 104 grams of sugar (that's the equivalent of 26 teaspoons) not to mention a good dose of artifical colours, flavours and preservatives. Consider yourself informed!

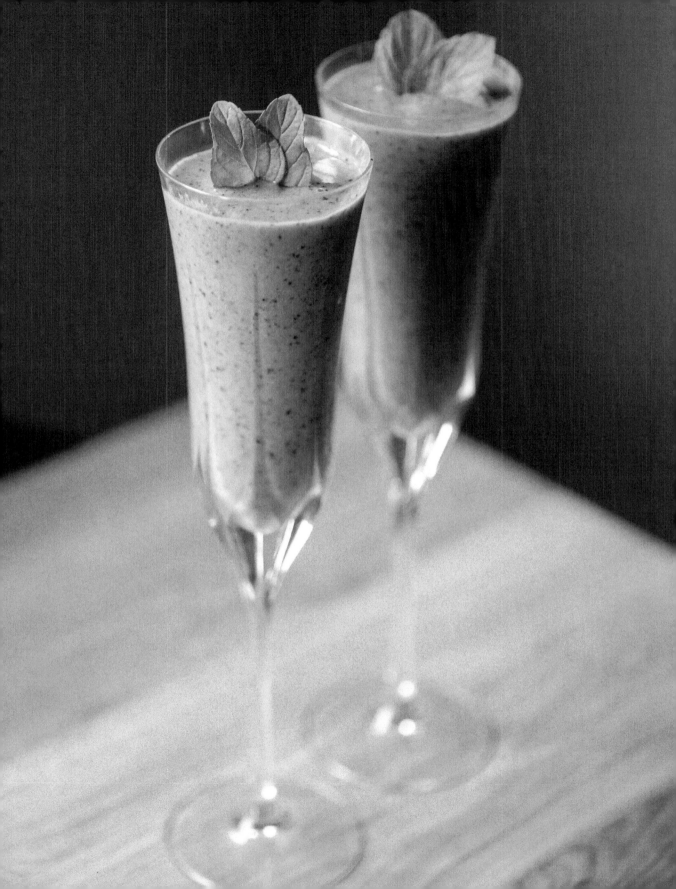

Berrylicious Smoothie

Serves 1

If you're looking for a delicious berry smoothie, then this is the drink for you! The berries provide anti-aging antioxidants and fibre, and the added nut butter and chia seeds provide an extra dose of healthy fats and protein.

INGREDIENTS:

- $1/2$ tablespoon ground chia seeds
- 1 cup nut or seed milk (I used hemp)
- 1 cup frozen mixed berries
- 1 tablespoon nut or seed butter (I used cashew-coconut butter)
- 1 frozen, ripe banana, chopped

INSTRUCTIONS:

1. Add all ingredients to a high-powered blender in the order listed and blend until smooth.
2. Serve immediately.

> **TIP:**
> Berries are naturally low in sugar and high in antioxidants and fiber so they are a great addition to a healthy diet. Unfortunately they are also high in pesticides when grown conventionally, so make sure to buy them organic.

Cacao-Goji Smoothie

Serves 1–2

This smoothie tastes just like a chocolate milkshake but is infused with a ton of superfoods that your cells are going to thank you for. Note that this smoothie is super filling and both calorie- and nutrient-dense, so it should be served as a meal rather than a snack.

INGREDIENTS:

- $1/2$ can chilled full-fat coconut milk (the milk, not the cream that rises to the top)
- $1/2$ frozen, ripe banana, chopped
- 1 cup unsweetened hemp milk
- 1 teaspoon lucuma powder
- 1 teaspoon maca powder
- 2 tablespoons goji berries
- 2 tablespoons raw cacao powder
- 2 tablespoons sunflower-seed butter
- 1 teaspoon pure vanilla extract

INSTRUCTIONS:

1. Add all ingredients to a high-powered blender in the order listed and blend until smooth.
2. Serve immediately.

> **TIP:**
> Gogi berries, also known as wolf berries, taste like a cross between a cranberry and strawberry. They are high in antioxidants and vitamin C, and are fantastic for naturally adding sweetness to beverages. Next time you make yourself a cup of tea, skip the sugar and throw in a few goji berries instead. Mmmmm...delicious and nutritious!

Basil-Pear Smoothie

Serves 1

The combination of refreshing basil and sweet pear makes this the perfect summer afternoon drink. Basil provides anti-inflammatory and anti-bacterial properties, and the pear adds a nice dose of fibre to keep you full longer.

INGREDIENTS:

- 1 large pear, chopped
- 3 fresh basil leaves
- 1 cup nut or seed milk (I used almond)
- 1 tablespoon raw honey
- juice of $^1/_2$ lime
- $^1/_2$ cup ice

INSTRUCTIONS:

1. Add all ingredients to a high-powered blender in the order listed and blend until smooth.
2. Serve immediately.

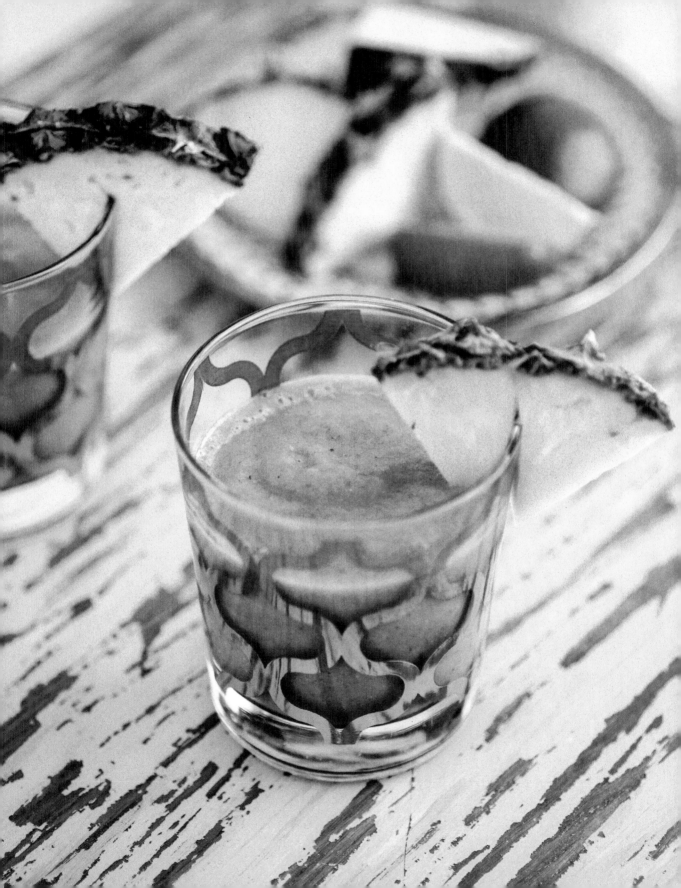

Pineapple Recovery Smoothie

Serves 1–2

If you feel like you need something to help you recover after an intense workout or hot yoga session, try this smoothie! The banana, celery, and coconut provide you with much-needed electrolytes that assist in rehydration. The pineapple and turmeric fight inflammation and are great for helping your muscles recuperate from a long sweat session.

INGREDIENTS:

- $1/2$ cup coconut water
- 1 cup frozen pineapple
- $1/2$ frozen, ripe banana, chopped
- 1 cup packed baby spinach
- 2 stalks celery
- 1 lime, peeled
- $1/2$ tablespoon ground flax seeds
- $1/2$ tablespoon ground chia seeds
- $1/2$ teaspoon ground turmeric
- $1/2$ teaspoon grated, peeled, fresh ginger
- $1/2$ cup ice

INSTRUCTIONS:

1. Add all ingredients to a high-powered blender in the order listed and blend until smooth.
2. Pour into a glass, sit back, and enjoy!

> TIP:
> Turmeric contains an active ingredient called curcumin, which is known for its strong anti-inflammatory effects, high levels of antioxidants and potent cancer-fighting properties. Curcumin is also available as a supplement in health food stores.

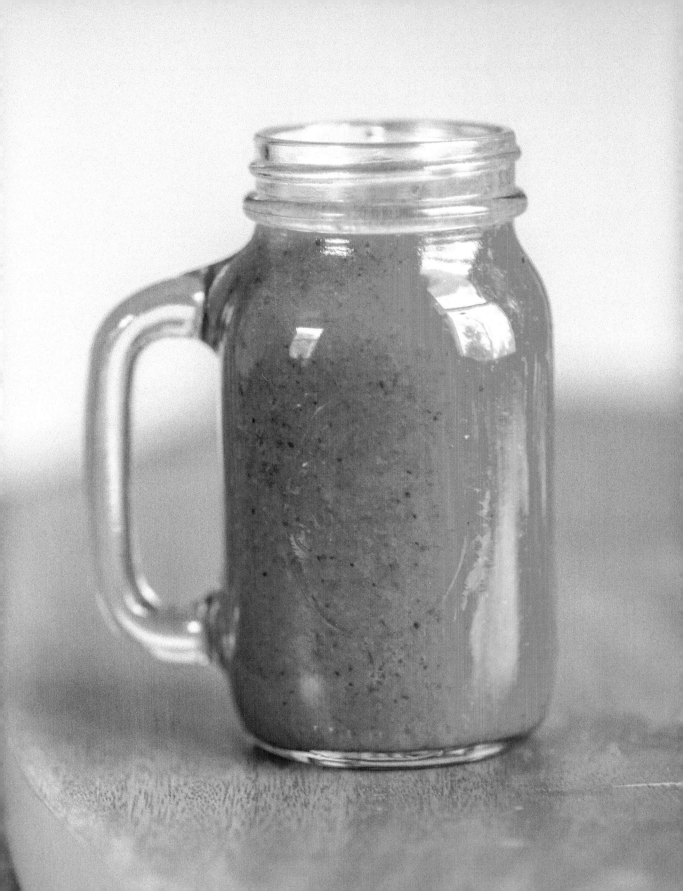

Can't-Be-Beet Smoothie

Serves 1–2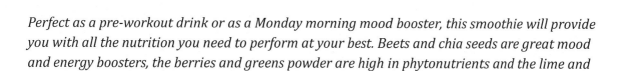

Perfect as a pre-workout drink or as a Monday morning mood booster, this smoothie will provide you with all the nutrition you need to perform at your best. Beets and chia seeds are great mood and energy boosters, the berries and greens powder are high in phytonutrients and the lime and orange juice are great sources of vitamin C. Oh, and did I mention that it tastes like a creamsicle?

INGREDIENTS:

- 1 cup freshly-squeezed orange juice
- $^1/_2$ cup unsweetened vanilla almond milk
- 1 small beet, peeled and chopped
- 1 cup frozen, mixed berries
- 1 scoop gluten-free greens powder
- juice of $^1/_2$ lime
- 1 tablespoon raw honey
- 1 tablespoon chia seeds
- $^1/_2$ cup ice

INSTRUCTIONS:

1. Add all ingredients to a high-powered blender in the order listed and blend until smooth.
2. Serve immediately.

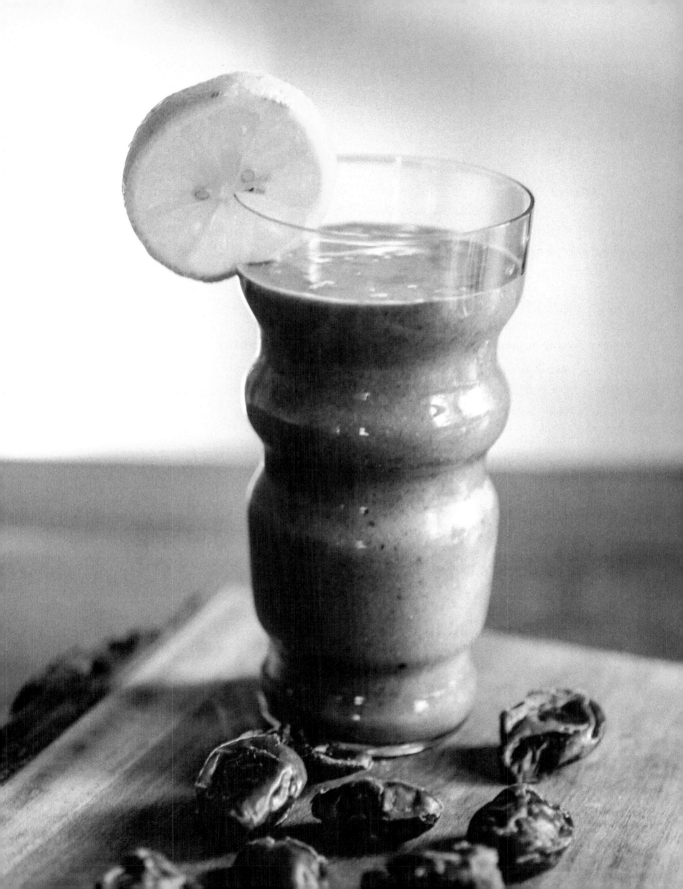

Strawberry-Peach Smoothie

Serves 1–2

There is just something magical that happens when you combine strawberries and peaches. Throw in some extra greens and a dose of vegan protein, and you have yourself a perfectly balanced, portable breakfast.

INGREDIENTS:

- 1 cup nut or seed milk
- $^1/_2$ cup water
- $^1/_2$ cup frozen strawberries
- $^1/_2$ cup frozen peaches
- 1 $^1/_2$ cups romaine lettuce
- a good squeeze of a lemon
- 2 pitted Medjool dates
- 2 tablespoons vegan protein powder
- $^1/_2$ scoop gluten-free greens powder
- 1 teaspoon pure vanilla extract
- $^1/_2$ cup ice

INSTRUCTIONS:

1. Add all ingredients to a high-powered blender in the order listed and blend until smooth.
2. Serve immediately.

TIP:

I like to use vegan protein powder quite often, but I also like to ensure that it is top quality and without any artificial sweeteners, colours or flavours. My favourite is the fermented vegan proteins+ powder by Genuine Health. Not only do they invest in independent third party testing for all of their products, but they are the only company to ferment their protein powder, making it gut-friendly and easier to digest. You can find it here: http://www.genuinehealth.com/store/fermented-vegan-proteins

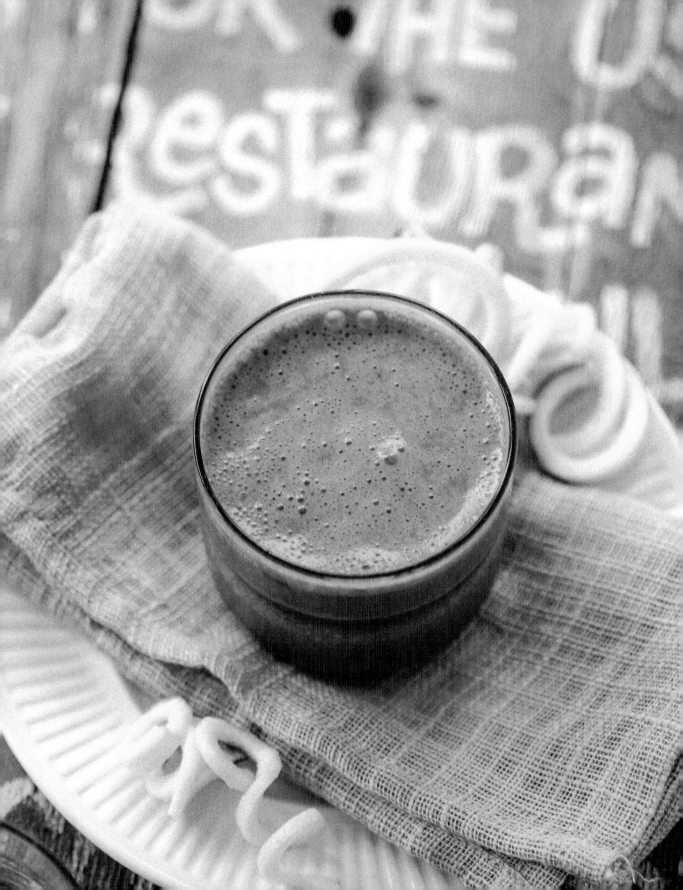

Chocolate Bliss Smoothie

Serves 1–2

Pure chocolate bliss! Those are the words that Marianne, my incredible food photographer, used when describing this smoothie, so I immediately named it after her suggestion. Trust me, you won't even be able to fathom that there is zucchini in there.

INGREDIENTS:

- 1 cup nut or seed milk (I like to use almond or hemp)
- 4 Brazil nuts
- 2 tablespoons raw cacao powder
- $1/2$ small zucchini, chopped
- 1 frozen, ripe banana, chopped
- 1 tablespoon almond butter
- 3 pitted Medjool dates
- a pinch of sea salt
- $1/2$ cup ice

INSTRUCTIONS:

1. Add all ingredients to a high-powered blender in the order listed and blend until smooth.
2. Serve immediately.

> TIP: 🍴
>
> Brazil nuts are also known as cream nuts due to their creamy and buttery taste and appearance. They also happen to be one of the highest natural sources of the mineral selenium, which is a critical factor for the proper functioning of our master antioxidant glutathione. Just 1-2 nuts a day ensures that you meet the Recommended Daily Amount (RDA) of this mineral. Brazil nuts are also an excellent source of B vitamins, which are needed for energy production and fighting stress, as well as a good source of vitamin E, which is another powerful antioxidant.

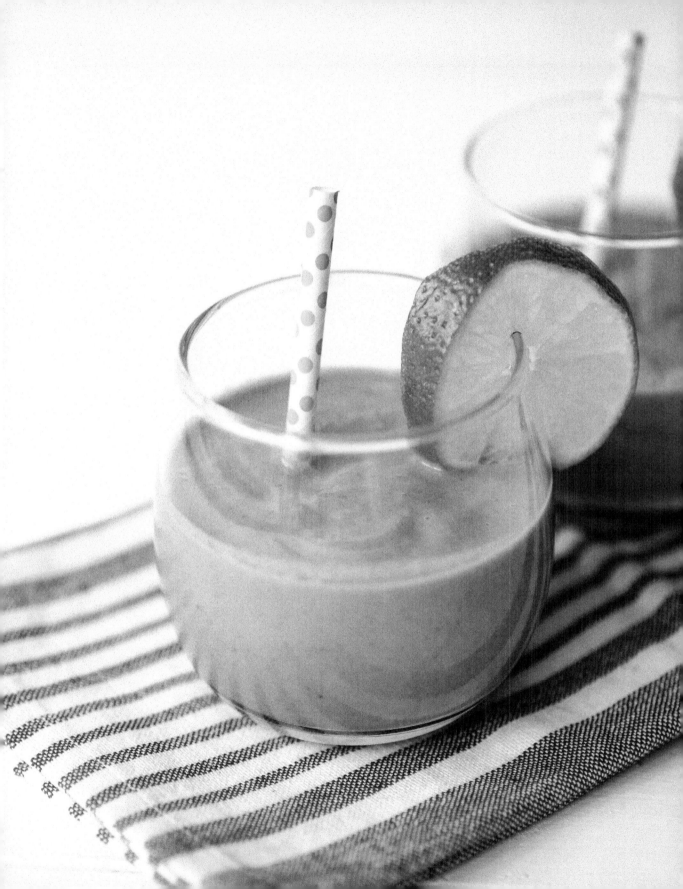

Mango-Peach Smoothie

Serves 1–2

The combination of these two fruits will make you feel like you're in the tropics, but because mangos and peaches are available in the freezer section of your grocery store year-round, you can easily enjoy this smoothie anytime of the year.

INGREDIENTS:

- 1 ¼ cups nut or seed milk
- 1 cup frozen mango
- ½ cup frozen peaches
- 2 pitted Medjool dates
- 1 cup baby spinach
- 1 teaspoon pure vanilla extract
- juice of 1 lime
- ½ cup ice

INSTRUCTIONS:

1. Add all ingredients to a high-powered blender in the order listed and blend until smooth.
2. Serve immediately.

TIP:
Don't let the colour of this smoothie scare you or your kids! It was an overwhelming favourite among our youngest taste-testers.

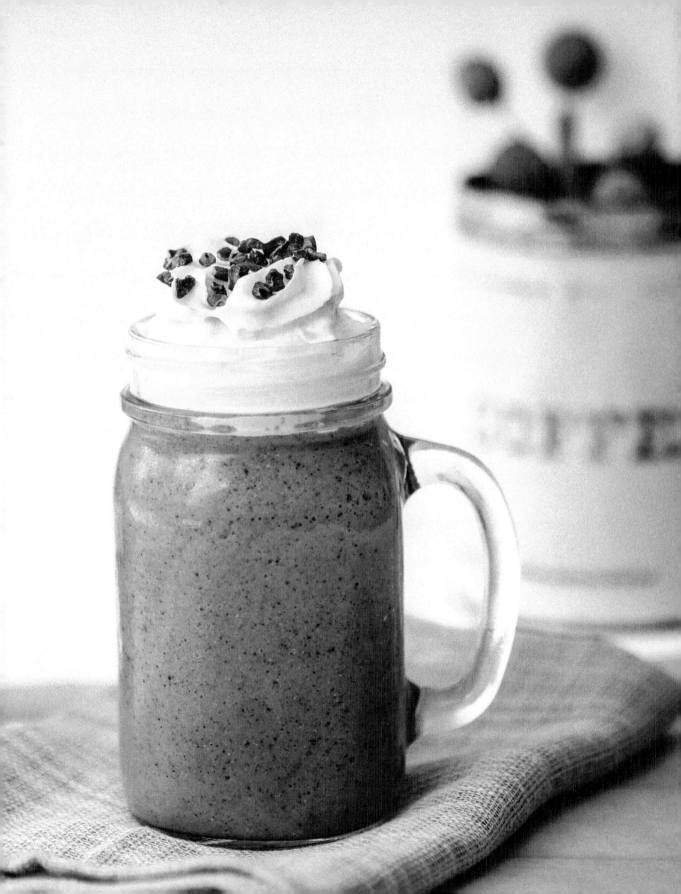

Java Chip Smoothie

Serves 1–2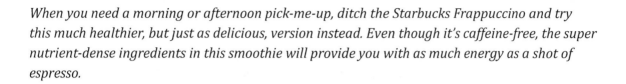

When you need a morning or afternoon pick-me-up, ditch the Starbucks Frappuccino and try this much healthier, but just as delicious, version instead. Even though it's caffeine-free, the super nutrient-dense ingredients in this smoothie will provide you with as much energy as a shot of espresso.

INGREDIENTS:

- 1 cup unsweetened almond milk
- 1 tablespoon Dandy Blend (or organic instant coffee)
- 1 $^1/_2$ tablespoons ground chia seeds
- 1 tablespoon almond butter
- 1 tablespoon real maple syrup
- 1 tablespoon raw cacao powder
- 2 pitted Medjool dates
- 1 teaspoon pure vanilla extract
- $^1/_4$–$^1/_2$ teaspoon ground cinnamon
- 20 large ice cubes
- topping: 1–2 teaspoons raw cacao nibs

INSTRUCTIONS:

1. Add all smoothie ingredients, with the exception of the cacao nibs, to a high-powered blender in the order listed, and blend until smooth.

2. Pour the smoothie into a large glass or mason jar. Drink by itself, or if desired, top with the *Coconut Whipped Cream* and *Chocolate Sauce* (from the *Sweet n' Savoury Dips and Dressings* section). Sprinkle with cacao nibs, and serve immediately.

> **TIP:** 🍴
>
> Although I love 'the bean' as much as anyone (just come by my house at 7 am and you will see!) caffeine has a half-life of 5–6 hours and some less than favourable outcomes for people who have trouble sleeping or who have high levels of the stress hormone, cortisol, coursing through their bodies (i.e. most of us). If you are one of those people, I recommend you try Dandy Blend, which is a gluten-free, caffeine-free, herbal beverage that tastes almost exactly like coffee, but without the bitterness. Look for it at your local health food store.

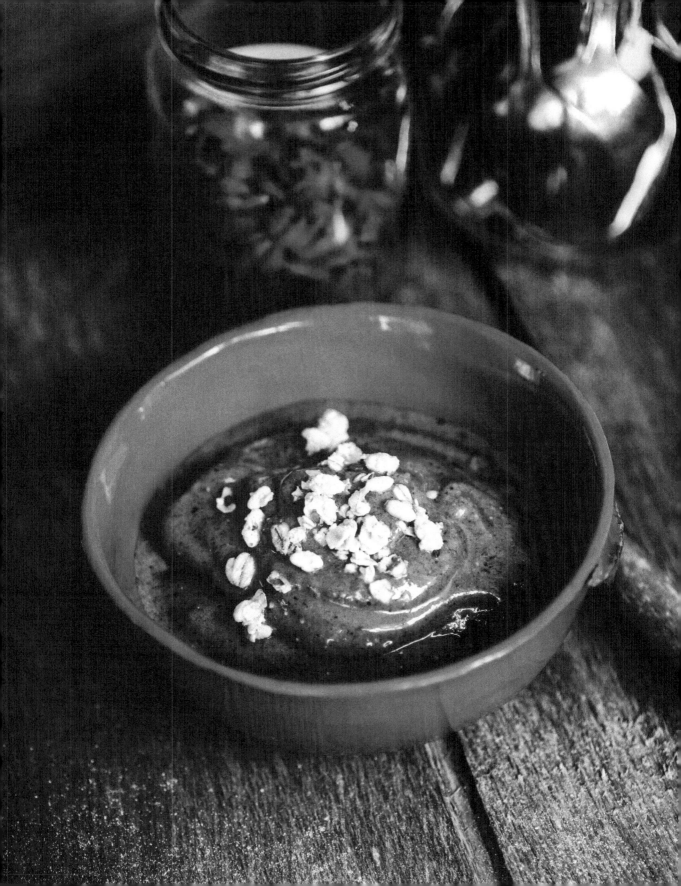

Raspberry-Banana Smoothie Bowl

Serves 2

I am so in love with smoothie bowls. They make me feel like I am eating a decadent dessert even though I am nourishing my body with nutrient-dense superfoods. This smoothie bowl is an excellent way to sneak in at least half of your daily recommended amount of fruits and veggies, and as a bonus, you get a mega dose of fibre.

INGREDIENTS:

- $^1/_2$ cup unsweetened hemp milk
- $^1/_4$ cup apple juice
- 1 frozen, ripe banana, chopped
- 1 cup frozen raspberries
- 3 cups baby spinach
- 1 tablespoon cashew butter
- 1 scoop (about $^1/_4$ cup) vanilla vegan protein powder
- 1 tablespoon dried goji berries
- 2 tablespoons shredded, unsweetened coconut
- $^1/_2$ cup ice
- topping: 2 tablespoons homemade granola

INSTRUCTIONS:

1. Add all ingredients, with the exception of the toppings, to a high-powered blender and blend until smooth. You may need to scrape down the sides of the blender a few times to get it moving. The smoothie should be extra thick.

2. Pour or ladle into a wide bowl and top with homemade granola (see below).

3. Eat immediately with a spoon.

TIP: Making homemade granola is super easy! Just mix together $^1/_8$ cup of melted coconut oil, $^1/_4$ cup maple syrup, 1 teaspoon vanilla and a pinch of sea salt. Pour over a mixture of 3 cups of gluten-free rolled oats, $^1/_2$ cup nuts, and $^1/_2$ cup seeds. Spread onto a baking sheet and bake at 300°F for 30 minutes or until golden brown.

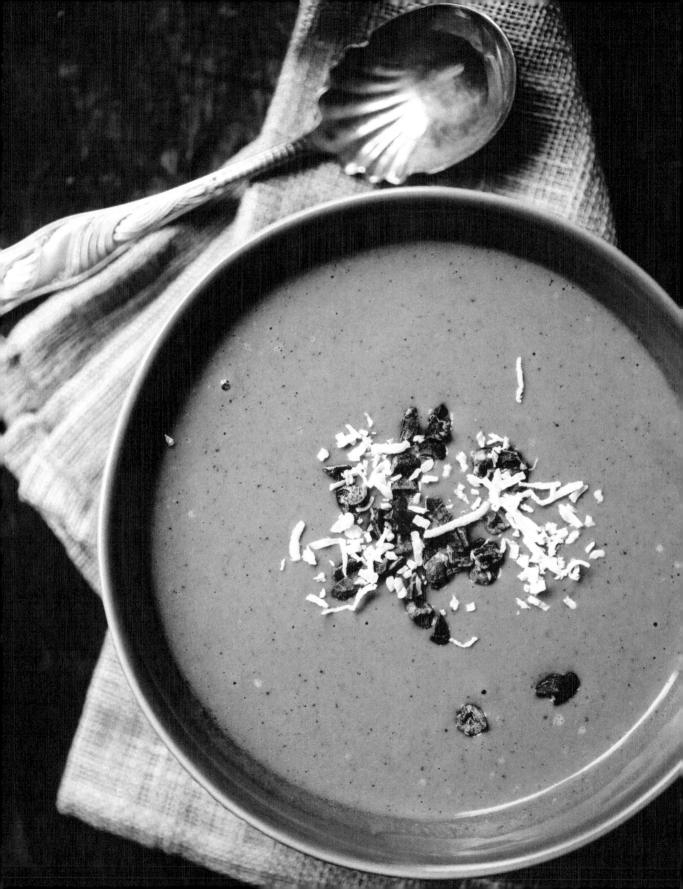

Mint-Chocolate-Chip Smoothie Bowl

Serves 2

This smoothie bowl, filled with three full cups of spinach, is a huge hit with all four of my kids because it tastes just like mint chocolate chip ice cream. Even better, each bowl contains good amounts of protein, iron, magnesium, zinc, folate, calcium, and vitamins A and K.

INGREDIENTS:

- $^2/_3$ cup unsweetened hemp milk
- 1 large frozen, ripe banana, chopped
- 3 cups baby spinach
- 1 tablespoon cashew butter
- 2–3 fresh mint leaves
- 1 scoop (about $^1/_4$ cup) vanilla vegan protein powder
- 2 tablespoons raw cacao nibs
- 1 pitted Medjool date
- 2 drops pure peppermint extract
- $^1/_2$ cup ice
- toppings: 1 tablespoon raw cacao nibs and 1 tablespoon shredded, unsweetened coconut, or 2 tablespoons homemade granola

INSTRUCTIONS:

1. Add all ingredients, with the exception of the toppings, to a high-powered blender and blend until smooth. You may need to scrape down the sides of the blender a few times to get it moving. The smoothie should be extra thick.

2. Pour or ladle into a wide bowl and top with cacao nibs and coconut, or homemade granola.

3. Eat immediately with a spoon. Swoon.

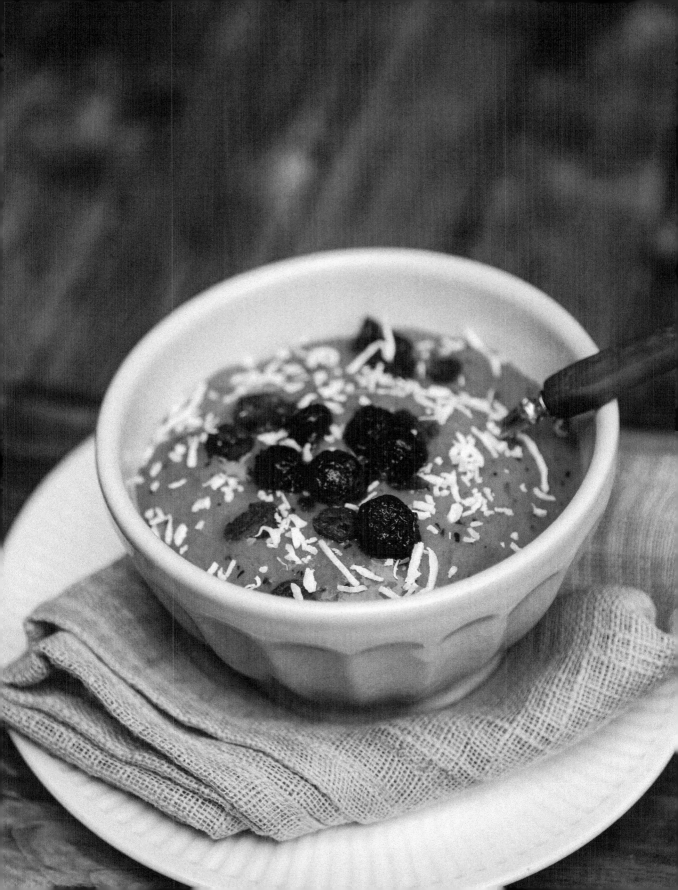

Strawberry-Plum Smoothie Bowl

Serves 2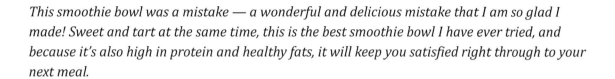

This smoothie bowl was a mistake — a wonderful and delicious mistake that I am so glad I made! Sweet and tart at the same time, this is the best smoothie bowl I have ever tried, and because it's also high in protein and healthy fats, it will keep you satisfied right through to your next meal.

INGREDIENTS:

- 1 cup unsweetened vanilla almond or coconut milk
- $^1/_2$ cup cold water
- 2 frozen, ripe bananas, chopped
- 4 plums, pitted and chopped
- 1 $^1/_4$ cups frozen strawberries
- 1 tablespoon almond butter
- 1 teaspoon maca powder
- 1 tablespoon ground chia/flax seed
- 1 scoop (about $^1/_4$ cup) vanilla vegan protein powder
- your favourite toppings

INSTRUCTIONS:

1. Add all ingredients, with the exception of the toppings, to a high-powered blender and blend until smooth. You may need to scrape down the sides of the blender a few times to get it moving. The smoothie should be extra thick.

2. Pour or ladle into a wide bowl and add your favourite toppings.

3. Eat immediately with a spoon. Double swoon.

> **TIP:**
> I recommend buying plums (and other fresh fruit) when they are in season and freezing them for future use. This way, you always have seasonal fruit on hand, and you save money at the same time. Win, win!

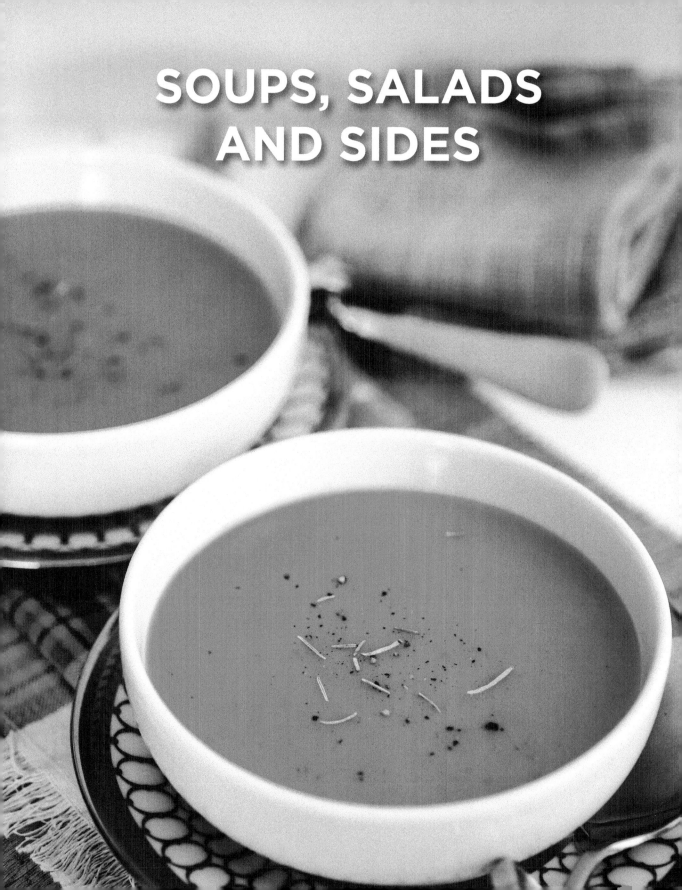

SOUPS, SALADS AND SIDES

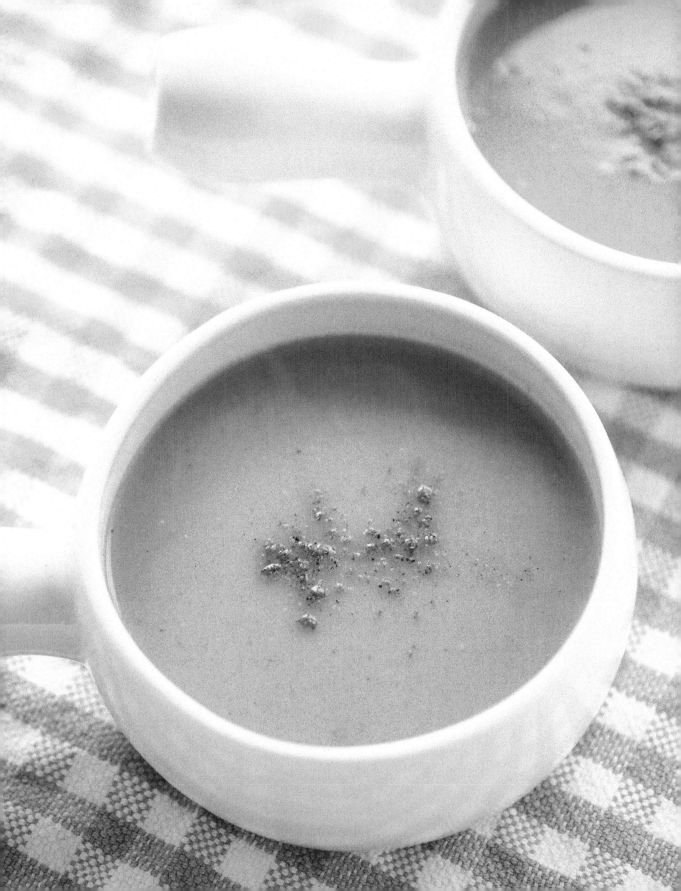

Butternut-Squash and Apple Soup

Serves 4-6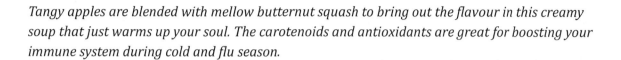

Tangy apples are blended with mellow butternut squash to bring out the flavour in this creamy soup that just warms up your soul. The carotenoids and antioxidants are great for boosting your immune system during cold and flu season.

INGREDIENTS:

- 1 large butternut squash
- 1 tablespoon coconut oil
- $^1/_4$ teaspoon sea salt
- 2 granny smith apples, peeled, seeded, and quartered
- 1 onion, peeled and quartered
- 2 cloves garlic, peeled
- $^1/_4$ cup water
- 6 cups chicken or vegetable broth
- 1 tablespoon minced, fresh ginger
- 1 teaspoon curry powder
- 1 teaspoon ground cinnamon
- $^1/_2$ teaspoon sea salt
- $^1/_4$ teaspoon freshly-ground pepper

INSTRUCTIONS:

1. Preheat oven to 350°F.

2. Cut the squash lengthwise and rub with coconut oil on the inside. Season with sea salt. Place face down onto a roasting pan. Add apples, onion, and garlic to the pan, pour in the water, and bake for 60 minutes or until squash can easily be pierced with a fork.

3. Remove the pan from the oven and let cool slightly, then scoop out the flesh from the squash and, together with apples, onion, and garlic, add to a large soup pot. Add in broth and spices and bring to a boil.

4. Reduce heat and simmer for ten minutes, then remove from heat and purée with an immersion blender until smooth.

5. Top with the *Roasted Chickpeas* (from this section) for a bit of added protein.

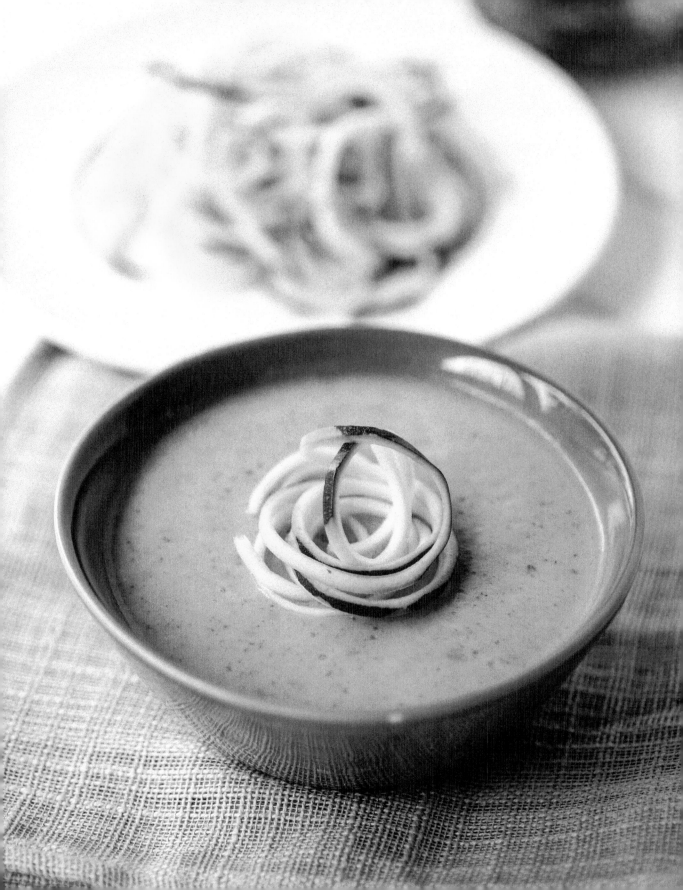

Creamy Zucchini Soup

Serves 4–6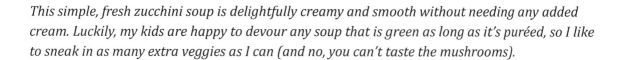

This simple, fresh zucchini soup is delightfully creamy and smooth without needing any added cream. Luckily, my kids are happy to devour any soup that is green as long as it's puréed, so I like to sneak in as many extra veggies as I can (and no, you can't taste the mushrooms).

INGREDIENTS:

- 1 tablespoon coconut oil
- $^1/_2$ medium onion, chopped
- 3 $^1/_2$ cups zucchini, chopped
- $^1/_2$ cup celery, chopped
- 1 cup carrots, peeled and chopped
- 1 cup mushrooms, sliced
- 4 cups chicken or vegetable broth
- 1 clove garlic, peeled and minced
- 1 potato, peeled and chopped
- 1 teaspoon dried marjoram
- $^1/_2$ teaspoon sea salt
- $^1/_4$ teaspoon freshly-ground pepper
- $^1/_4$ cup fresh parsley, chopped

INSTRUCTIONS:

1. Melt the coconut oil in a large pot. Sauté onion, zucchini, celery, carrots, and mushrooms until softened, about ten minutes, adding a tiny bit of water if the vegetables start to stick.

2. Add chicken broth, garlic, potato, marjoram, sea salt, and ground pepper, and boil for ten more minutes, then remove from heat and purée with an immersion blender until smooth.

3. Top with parsley right before serving.

TIP:

Low in calories and carbohydrates, high in nutrients, smooth in texture, and mild in flavour, zucchinis are incredibly versatile. For example, you can sneak them into meatballs unnoticed and they make a great substitute for pasta! Simply spiralize them using a spiralizer, sauté them in coconut oil for a few minutes and top with your regular pasta sauce.

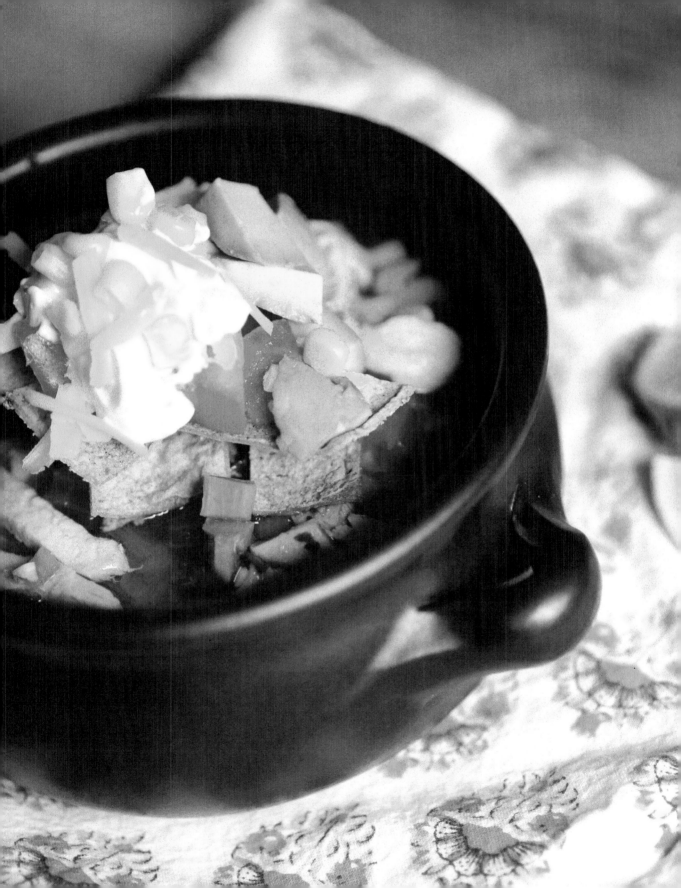

Chicken Tortilla Soup

Serves 6-8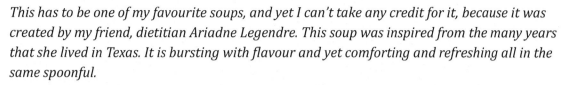

This has to be one of my favourite soups, and yet I can't take any credit for it, because it was created by my friend, dietitian Ariadne Legendre. This soup was inspired from the many years that she lived in Texas. It is bursting with flavour and yet comforting and refreshing all in the same spoonful.

INGREDIENTS:

- 4 gluten-free tortillas
- sea salt, to taste
- 1 tablespoon coconut oil
- 3 cloves garlic, peeled and finely chopped
- 1 medium onion, peeled and finely chopped
- 2 medium carrots, chopped in small pieces
- 2 stalks celery, chopped in small pieces
- 1 jalapeño, seeded and finely chopped
- 2 cups diced tomatoes
- 1 cup of corn kernels (fresh or frozen)
- 6 cups chicken broth
- 2 tablespoons of ground cumin
- 1 teaspoon of dried oregano
- 2 cups of cooked, shredded chicken
- a handful of fresh cilantro, finely chopped
- sea salt and freshly-ground pepper, to taste
- optional toppings: avocado slices, fresh lime juice, fresh cilantro, freshly diced tomatoes

INSTRUCTIONS:

1. Preheat the oven to 375°F. Cut the tortillas into thin strips and sprinkle with salt. Arrange the tortilla strips into a single layer on a baking sheet. Bake in the oven for a few minutes until light brown and crisp, but watch them carefully as they can burn quickly. Set aside to cool.

2. In a large saucepan, heat the oil at medium-high temperature. Add the garlic, onions, carrots, celery, and jalapeños, and sauté until tender (about 3–5 minutes).

3. Add the tomatoes, corn, chicken stock, cumin, and oregano and simmer for approximately 30 minutes or until the vegetables are tender.

4. Add the chicken and cilantro and let simmer another 5–10 minutes.

5. Ladle the soup into bowls. Top each serving with a little nest of tortilla strips and optional toppings if using.

> **TIP:** 🍴
> If you prefer, feel free to skip step #1 and use organic tortilla chips instead of the gluten-free tortillas. Simply crush the tortilla chips and sprinkle them on top of the cooked soup before serving for an added bit of crunch.

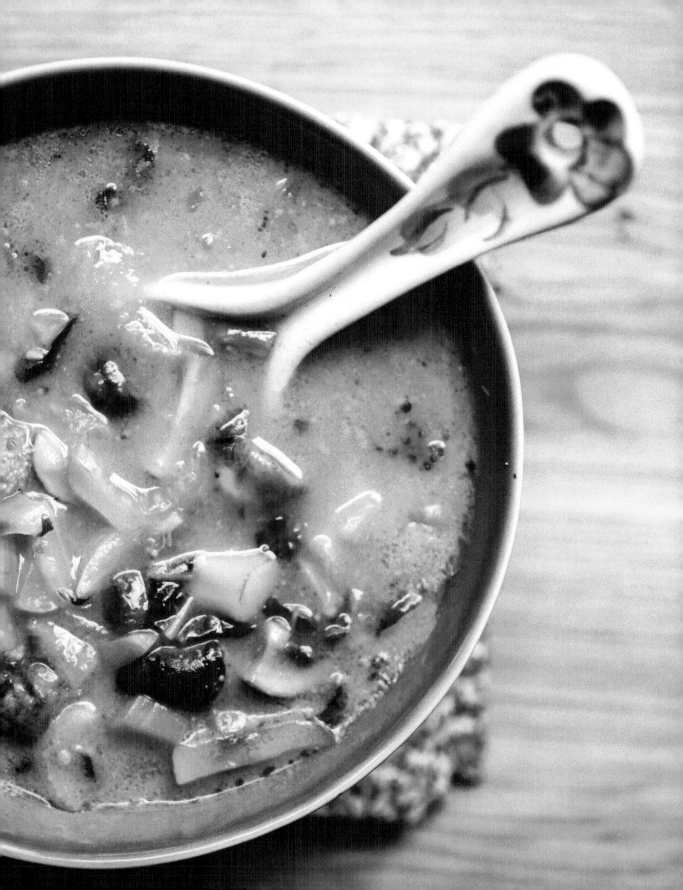

Thai Coconut Soup

Serves 4-6

The soup is so mind-blowingly delicious and its flavours are so complex that you almost forget that it's actually good for you. Combined with its great immune-boosting and detoxifying powers, you will want to make this soup over and over again.

INGREDIENTS:

- 1 tablespoon coconut oil
- $1/2$ cup red onion, peeled and chopped
- 1 cup Chinese cabbage, shredded
- 2 carrots, peeled and sliced
- 1 cup cremini mushrooms, chopped
- 3 broccoli stalks, chopped
- 6 cups homemade chicken or vegetable broth
- 2 tablespoons grated, fresh ginger
- 1 stalk lemongrass, shredded
- 2 tablespoons red chili paste
- 2 tablespoons fresh tamari
- 2 tablespoons organic miso paste
- 3 tablespoons freshly-squeezed lemon juice
- $1/2$ cup dried dulse, chopped
- $1/2$ can full-fat coconut milk
- 1 tablespoon raw honey
- $1/2$ cup fresh cilantro leaves, chopped

INSTRUCTIONS:

1. Melt oil in a large soup pot over medium heat. Add the onion and sauté a few minutes until translucent. Add cabbage, carrots, cremini mushrooms, and broccoli stalks, and sauté a few more minutes. Add broth, ginger, lemongrass, chili paste, tamari, miso paste, lemon juice, and dulse, and bring to a boil.

2. Once boiling, reduce heat and simmer for 20–30 minutes or until all vegetables are cooked through. Remove from heat and add in coconut milk, honey, and fresh cilantro.

3. Serve warm.

TIP:

Tamari is a fermented soy sauce that is usually gluten-free (check the label to make sure). I personally prefer to cook with tamari as it's smoother, less salty, and has more depth than regular soy sauce. It's also high in niacin, manganese, protein, and tryptophan. Make sure to buy the organic version, as most conventionally-grown soy beans are genetically modified.

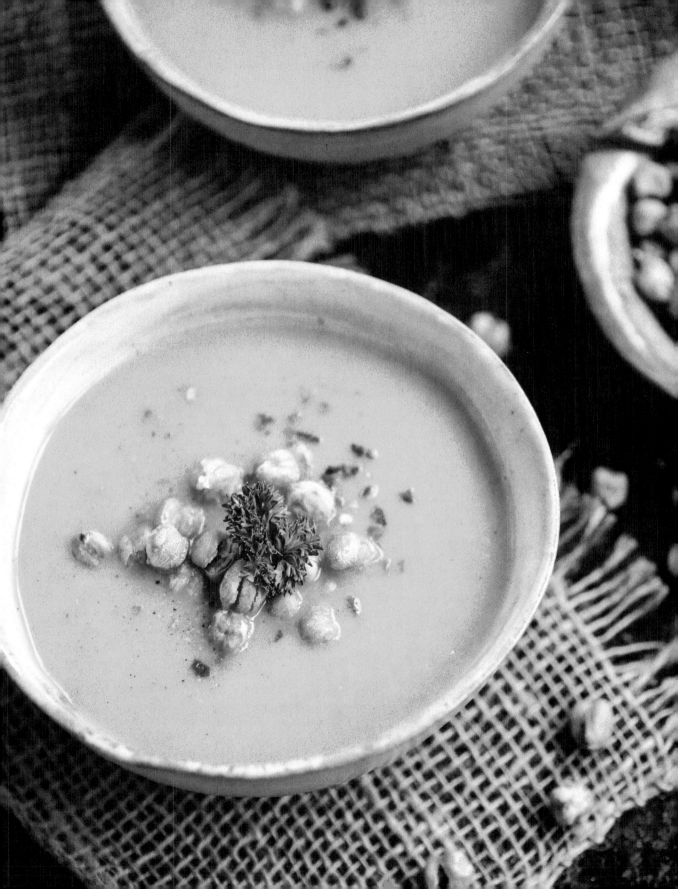

Carrot, Orange, and Ginger Soup

Serves 6-8

Spicy and sweet, this soup is the ideal comfort food for spring and fall months. High in anti-inflammatory properties, easy on digestion, and filled with beta-carotene and vitamin C, this soup will help keep you strong, healthy, and vibrant.

INGREDIENTS:

- 1 tablespoon coconut oil
- 1 medium yellow onion, peeled and chopped
- 7–8 large carrots, peeled and chopped
- 1 tablespoon grated, fresh ginger
- 1 clove garlic, crushed
- 6 cups chicken or vegetable broth
- a splash of sesame oil
- 1 cup freshly-squeezed orange juice
- 1 tablespoon raw honey
- 1 tablespoon curry power
- $1/2$ teaspoon ground cinnamon
- 1 teaspoon sea salt
- $1/4$ teaspoon freshly-ground black pepper
- toppings: a sprinkle of red pepper flakes and $1/4$ cup fresh parsley

INSTRUCTIONS:

1. Melt coconut oil in a large pot over medium heat. Add onions and sauté until translucent.

2. Add carrots, ginger, garlic, and chicken stock. Bring to a boil, reduce heat, and let simmer for about 25-30 minutes or until carrots are tender.

3. When soup has finished cooking for the above-noted time, add in sesame oil, orange juice, honey, curry powder, cinnamon, salt, and pepper, and then remove from heat.

4. Use an immersion blender to purée soup until smooth.

5. Top with red pepper flakes, fresh parsley, and *Roasted Chickpeas* (from this section) if desired.

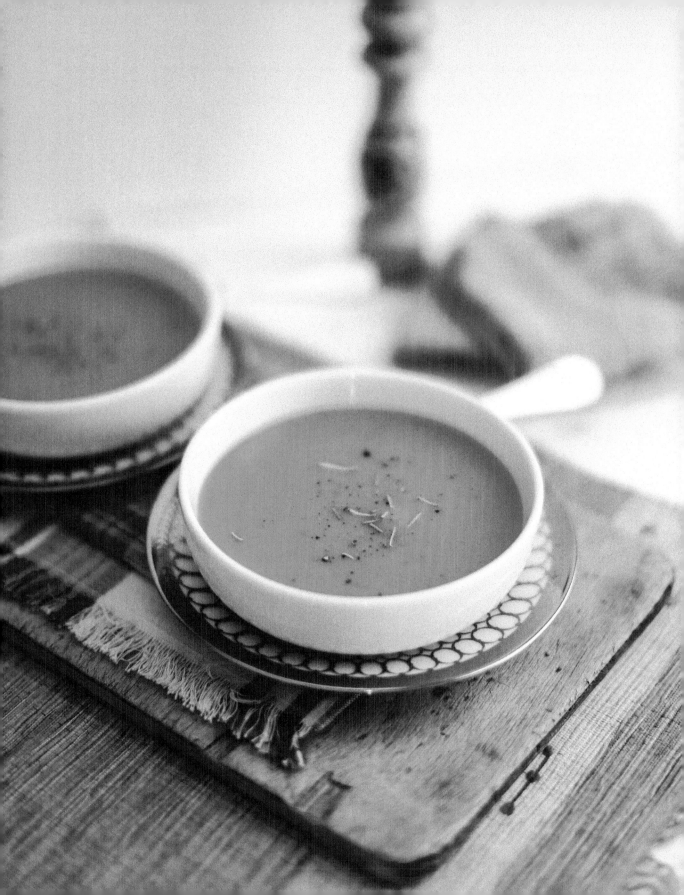

Roasted Red-Pepper Soup

Serves 4–6

This roasted red pepper soup is sweet, fresh, and earthy, and is low in calories but high in satiety. Red peppers are incredibly high in vitamin C and cancer-fighting properties and carrots are high in beta-carotene, which is a potent antioxidant. Serve it alongside a toasted gluten-free baguette.

INGREDIENTS:

- 2 red bell peppers, seeded and halved
- 1 tablespoon coconut oil
- 1 large sweet onion, peeled and chopped
- 2 carrots, peeled and chopped
- 1 potato, peeled and chopped
- 1 garlic clove, crushed
- $^1/_2$ cup dry white wine
- 4 cups chicken or vegetable broth
- 1 teaspoon dried thyme
- 1 teaspoon dried rosemary
- 1 teaspoon sea salt

INSTRUCTIONS:

1. Preheat oven to 400°F.
2. Place the peppers, skin-side-up, on a baking sheet near the top of the oven and roast for 20–30 minutes, until the skin starts to blacken.
3. Remove peppers from the oven and let cool, then peel off skin, and chop into small pieces.
4. In a medium-sized saucepan, sauté onion in coconut oil until translucent.
5. Add in carrots and sauté for another two minutes.
6. Add in the potatoes, garlic, roasted red peppers, white wine, chicken broth, and seasonings, and cook for another 20 minutes, partially covered.
7. Remove from heat and purée with an immersion blender until smooth.
8. Serve with a gluten-free baguette or top with some *Roasted Chickpeas* (from this section).

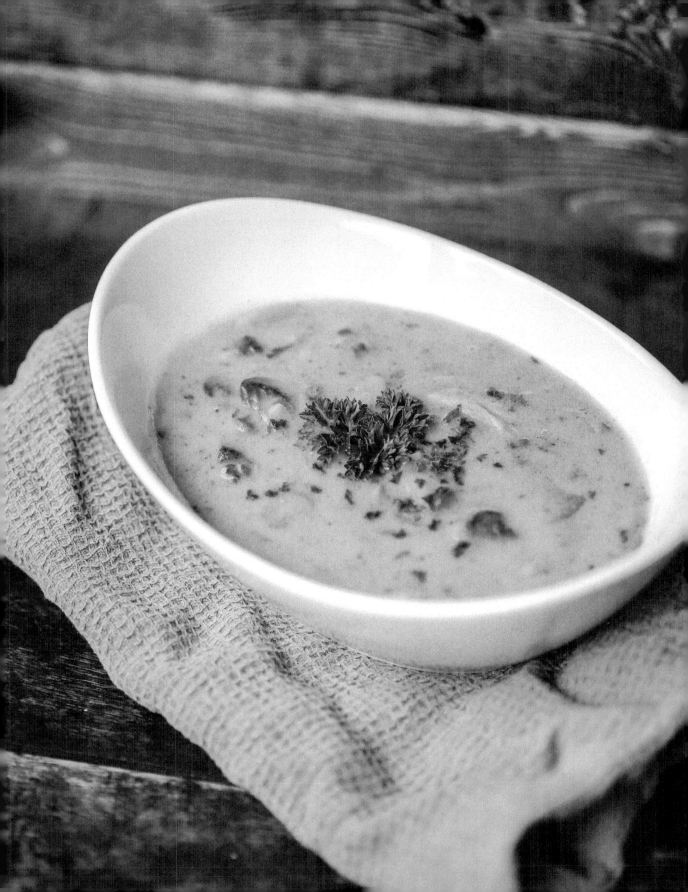

Creamy Mushroom Soup

Serves 4–6

You'll love this cream of mushroom soup, that has no cream, yet is just as creamy and delicious! Mushrooms are potent cancer-fighters and rich in almost all B vitamins, which are great for fighting the negative effects of stress and boosting your energy levels. Mushrooms are also rich in selenium, a powerful antioxidant, making this soup your secret immune defense.

INGREDIENTS:

- 1 tablespoon extra-virgin olive oil
- 1 onion, peeled and chopped
- 3 $\frac{1}{2}$ cups cremini mushrooms, chopped
- 2 tablespoons gluten-free flour mix or 1 potato, peeled and finely chopped
- 6 cups chicken or vegetable broth
- $\frac{1}{2}$ teaspoon ground nutmeg
- sea salt and freshly-ground pepper, to taste
- optional: 1–2 tablespoons coconut cream
- fresh parsley, for garnish

INSTRUCTIONS:

1. In a medium saucepan, sauté onion in olive oil until translucent.
2. Add in the mushrooms and cook for another three minutes. Reserve a half cup of mushrooms for garnish.
3. Add in the gluten-free flour (or potato) and sauté for two more minutes.
4. Add in chicken stock and bring to a boil.
5. Reduce heat and simmer for 20 minutes (or until potato is cooked through).
6. Add in nutmeg, salt, and pepper, and simmer for one more minute.
7. Remove from heat, add in coconut cream if desired, and purée with an immersion blender until smooth.
8. Garnish with reserved mushrooms and fresh parsley.

TIP:
Use this soup as the base for the *Healthy Shepherd's Pie* in the *Entrées* section.

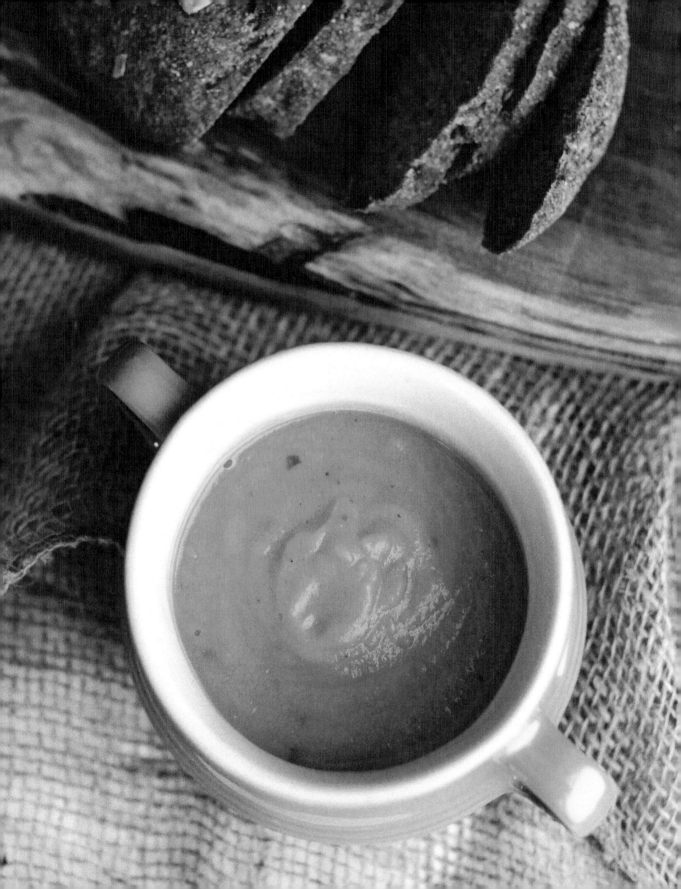

Creamy Tomato Soup

Serves 4–5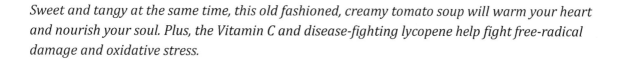

Sweet and tangy at the same time, this old fashioned, creamy tomato soup will warm your heart and nourish your soul. Plus, the Vitamin C and disease-fighting lycopene help fight free-radical damage and oxidative stress.

INGREDIENTS:

- 1 tablespoon extra-virgin olive oil
- 1 onion, peeled, chopped, and diced
- 2 carrots, peeled and grated
- 1 (28-ounce) can diced tomatoes or 5 fresh vine-ripened tomatoes, chopped
- 3 cups water
- 1 potato, peeled and chopped
- 2 bay leaves
- 1 teaspoon dried basil
- 1 teaspoon dried oregano
- 1–2 cloves crushed garlic
- sea salt and freshly-ground pepper, to taste
- $1/4$ cup chopped fresh parsley

INSTRUCTIONS:

1. In a medium saucepan, sauté onion in olive oil until translucent.
2. Add in carrots and sauté for another two minutes.
3. Add in the tomatoes and cook for another ten minutes, partially covered.
4. Add water, potato and bay leaf, cover and simmer for 15 more minutes.
5. Remove from heat and remove the bay leaf, then purée with an immersion blender until smooth.
6. Place back onto the heat and add in herbs, garlic, salt, and pepper.
7. Cook five more minutes, then remove from heat and add in fresh parsley.
8. Serve immediately.

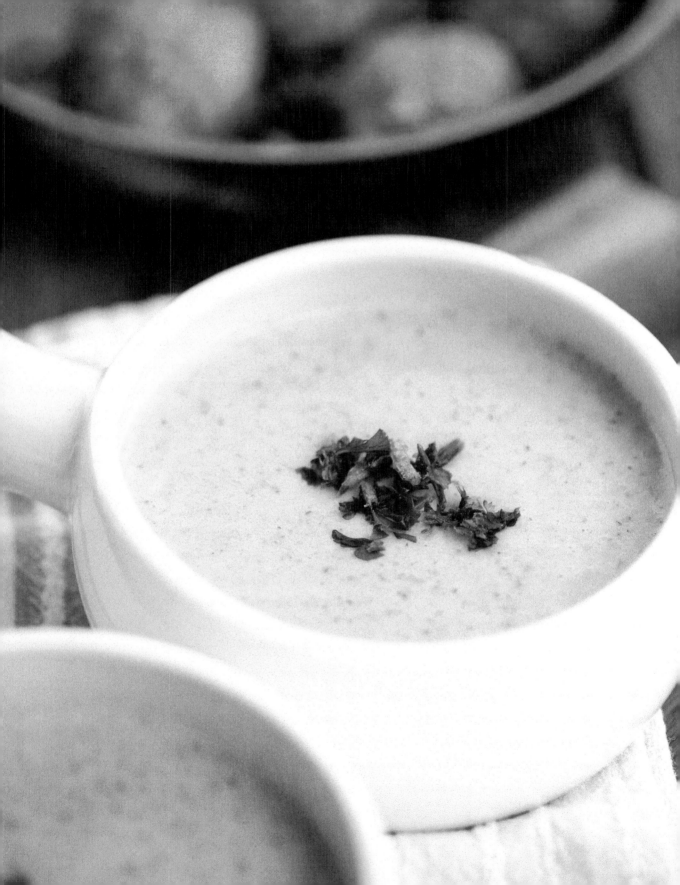

Cheesy Broccoli Soup

Serves 4-6

I used to love cheesy broccoli soup as a kid and missed it immensely when I gave up dairy — until I came up with this amazing recipe. Low in fat, loaded with calcium, and high in cancer-fighting properties, this creamy soup is the perfect ending for a cool autumn's day.

INGREDIENTS:

Sauce ingredients:

- 1 cup unsweetened almond or coconut milk
- $3/4$ cup nutritional yeast
- 1 tablespoon Dijon mustard
- 1 tablespoon freshly-squeezed lemon juice
- $1/2$ teaspoon sea salt
- 2 tablespoons cashew butter

Soup ingredients:

- 1 tablespoon coconut oil
- 1 onion, peeled and chopped
- 2 stalks celery, chopped
- 1 potato, peeled and chopped
- 3 cups broccoli florets
- 1 teaspoon minced garlic
- 3 cups chicken or vegetable broth

INSTRUCTIONS:

1. To make the sauce, warm up the almond milk in a small pot over medium heat. Once the milk is hot, but not boiling, add in nutritional yeast, Dijon, lemon juice, sea salt, and cashew butter, and whisk until well blended.

2. To make soup, in a medium saucepan, sauté onion and celery in coconut oil over medium heat until translucent. Add potato, broccoli, and garlic, and sauté for another minute. Add in broth and bring to a boil.

3. Lower heat to a simmer and cook for 20 minutes or until potato is cooked through.

4. Remove from heat and use an immersion blender to purée soup until smooth. Whisk the cheesy sauce into the soup and serve.

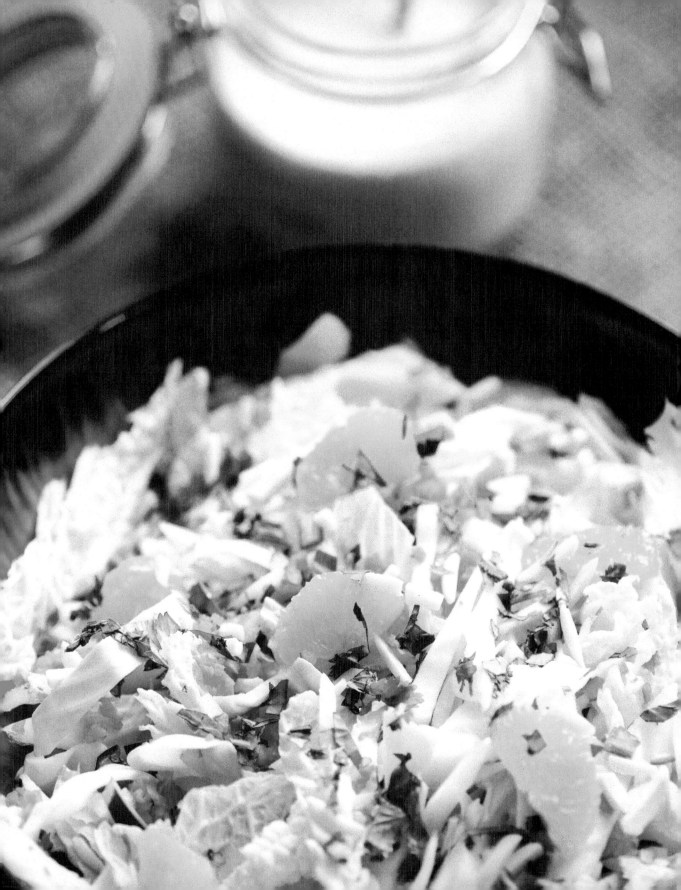

Sweet Cabbage Salad

Serves 4-6

This colourful, crunchy salad pairs wonderfully with the Creamy Dreamy Miso Dressing for an incredibly tasty meal! The cabbage is a potent cancer-fighter, the cilantro is a potent detoxifyer, the almonds are high in calcium and protein, and the carrots and oranges are high in antioxidants, making this salad a nutritional powerhouse!

INGREDIENTS:

- $^1/_2$ head each, of Napa cabbage, green cabbage, and red cabbage, thinly sliced
- 1 cup peeled, shredded carrots
- $^1/_4$ cup red onion, peeled and finely chopped
- $^3/_4$ cup fresh cilantro leaves, chopped
- $^1/_4$ cup slivered almonds
- 2 mandarin oranges, peeled and separated, or 1 mango, sliced

INSTRUCTIONS:

1. To make salad, mix all salad ingredients together in a large bowl.
2. Serve with *Creamy Miso Dressing* (from the *Sweet n' Savoury Dips and Dressings* section).

> **TIP:**
> Cabbage is high in fiber, sulfur, and vitamins K, C, and B6. It's ideal for weight loss because it's low in fat and high in fiber, and it's amazingly alkalizing and detoxifying. Cabbage juice is also great for reducing hangovers and minimizing headaches.

California Salad

Serves 4-6

A new take on the traditional California salad, the delicious contrast of flavours and textures makes this a salad you will want to make over and over again. The creamy avocado, crunchy seeds, and steamed veggies add depth and increase its nutritional profile, so it can easily be served as a main meal.

INGREDIENTS:

- ¹/₄ cup asparagus, chopped into pieces
- ¹/₄ cup green sweet peas
- ¹/₄ cup cauliflower florets, broken into tiny pieces
- 6 cups chopped romaine lettuce
- 1 avocado, peeled and sliced
- 1 tablespoon sunflower seeds
- 1 tablespoon pumpkin seeds
- 1 tablespoon hemp hearts

INSTRUCTIONS:

1. To make the salad, steam asparagus, green peas, and cauliflower in a steamer basket over boiling water for about two minutes, and then cool immediately under cold-running water.

2. Place the romaine lettuce in a large bowl and top with steamed veggies and seeds.

3. Top with avocado slices and serve with the *Maple Dijon Dressing* (from the *Sweet n' Savoury Dips and Dressings* section).

TIP:

Hemp hearts are high in protein and contain the perfect balance of omega-3's and omega-6's. Throw them in smoothies and salads, use them to make creamy dips and dressings, and add them into cookies and granolas for added crunch and texture.

Late-Summer Cabbage Salad

Serves 4–6

Cool, crunchy, and refreshingly light, the addition of fresh blueberries make this the perfect salad for summer days and, because of its sweet flavours, even kids will eat it. High in fibre, antioxidants, and sulphur-containing compounds, this salad is a potent cancer-fighter, anti-aging agent, immune booster, and detoxifier.

INGREDIENTS:

Salad ingredients:

- 1 $^1/_2$ cups green cabbage, thinly sliced
- 1 $^1/_2$ cups red cabbage, thinly sliced
- 2 medium carrots, peeled and shredded
- 1 medium beet, peeled and shredded
- 1 medium apple, peeled and shredded

Topping ingredients:

- 1 cup blueberries (or more to taste)
- 2 tablespoons hemp hearts
- 2 tablespoons sunflower seeds

INSTRUCTIONS:

1. To make salad, mix all salad ingredients together in a large bowl and set aside.
2. Sprinkle with toppings, and serve with the *Apple-Cider Vinaigrette* (from the *Sweet n' Savoury Dips and Dressings* section).

> **TIP:**
> To save time, use the shredding attachment of your food processor to shred the carrots, beet, and apple, and the slicing attachment for slicing the cabbage.

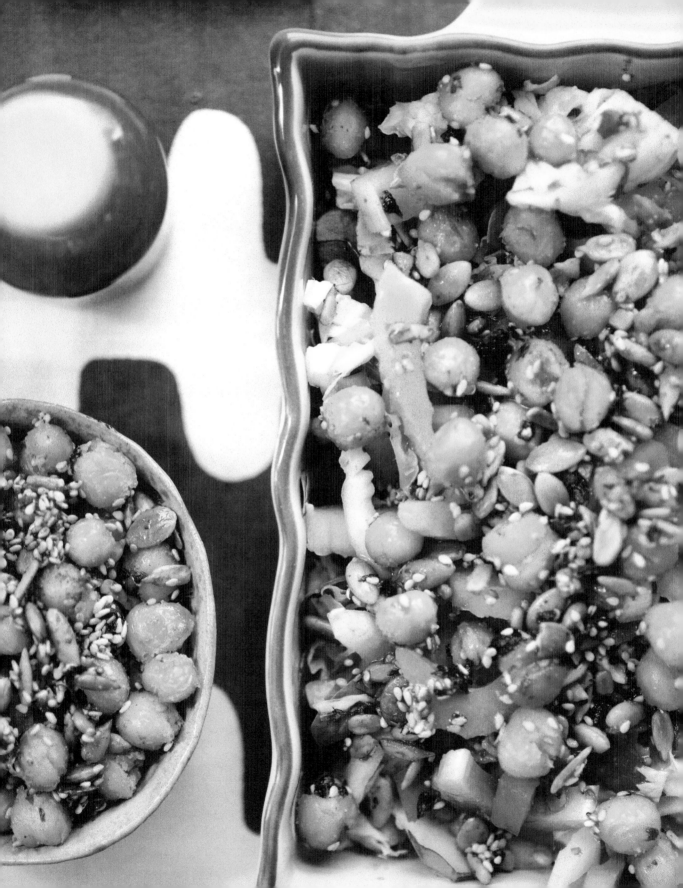

Seeduction Salad

Serves 4–6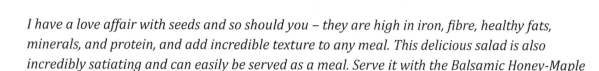

I have a love affair with seeds and so should you – they are high in iron, fibre, healthy fats, minerals, and protein, and add incredible texture to any meal. This delicious salad is also incredibly satiating and can easily be served as a meal. Serve it with the Balsamic Honey-Maple dressing for a true taste sensation!

INGREDIENTS:

Topping ingredients:

- 1 (14-ounce) can organic chickpeas, rinsed, drained and patted dry
- 1 teaspoon ground cumin
- 1 teaspoon garlic powder
- $1/2$ teaspoon ground coriander
- $1/4$ teaspoon cayenne pepper
- $1/4$ teaspoon sea salt
- 2 tablespoons coconut oil, melted
- 3 tablespoons sesame seeds
- 3 tablespoons pumpkin seeds
- 3 tablespoons sunflower seeds

Salad ingredients:

- 3 cups baby spinach
- 3 cups Napa cabbage, finely sliced
- 1 celery stalk, chopped into small pieces
- $1/4$ large red bell pepper, chopped into small pieces

INSTRUCTIONS:

1. Mix together all topping ingredients, with the exception of the coconut oil and the seeds, in a large bowl.

2. Heat coconut oil in a pan over medium heat. Once melted, add in the chickpea mixture and sauté for about 4–5 minutes over medium-high heat. Add in the seeds and saute for another 1–2 minutes. Remove and let cool.

3. To make salad, mix together all salad ingredients in a large bowl.

4. Sprinkle topping over salad, and drizzle with *Balsamic Honey-Maple Dressing* (from the *Sweet n' Savoury Dips and Dressings* section).

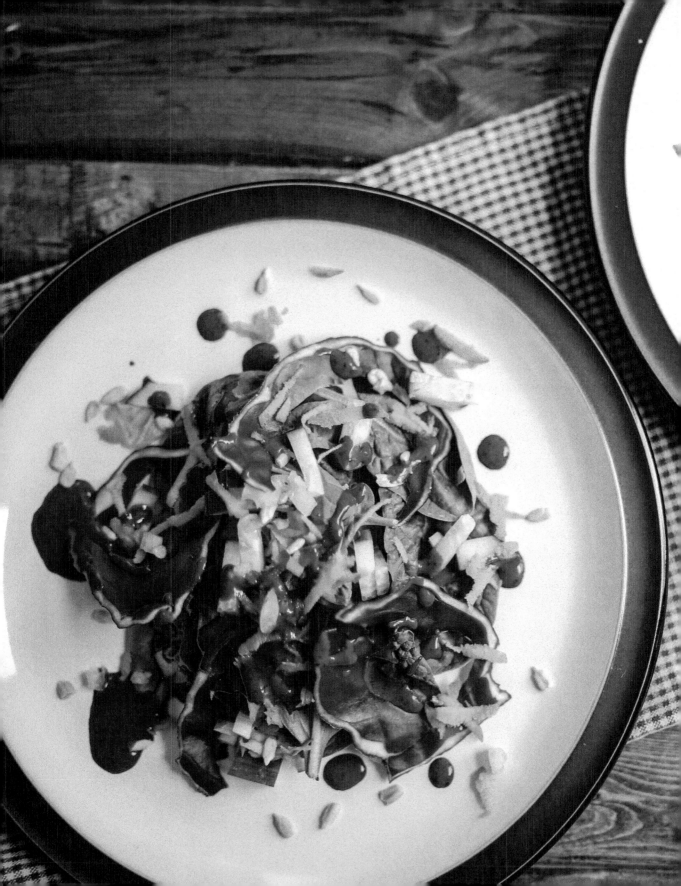

Sweet Beet-Carrot-Apple Salad

Serves 4–6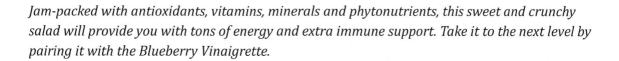

Jam-packed with antioxidants, vitamins, minerals and phytonutrients, this sweet and crunchy salad will provide you with tons of energy and extra immune support. Take it to the next level by pairing it with the Blueberry Vinaigrette.

INGREDIENTS:

- 6 cups baby spinach or romaine lettuce
- 2 carrots, peeled and grated
- 1 cup red cabbage, thinly sliced
- 1 small beet, peeled and grated
- 1 granny smith apple, peeled and grated
- 1 Lebanese cucumber, chopped (or $^1/_2$ regular cucumber, chopped)
- $^1/_2$ cup jicama, peeled and diced
- topping: 2–3 tablespoons nuts and seeds of your choice

INSTRUCTIONS:

1. Mix together all salad ingredients in a large bowl.
2. Top with nuts and seeds, and drizzle with the *Blueberry Vinaigrette* (from the *Sweet n' Savoury Dips and Dressings* section).

> **TIP:** 🍴
> Jicama is an edible root that resembles a turnip and tastes like a savoury apple. If you've never tried it, now's the time because it's absolutely delicous! Sweet, juicy, and crunchy, jicamas and kohlorabis are two of my favourite vegetables on this planet.

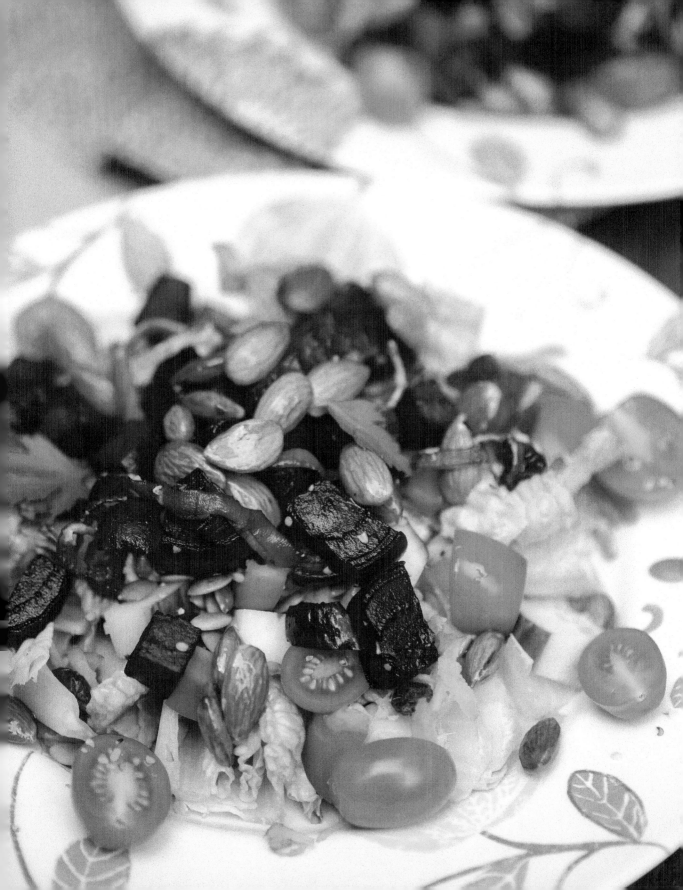

Roasted Beet Salad

Serves 4-6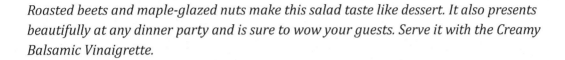

Roasted beets and maple-glazed nuts make this salad taste like dessert. It also presents beautifully at any dinner party and is sure to wow your guests. Serve it with the Creamy Balsamic Vinaigrette.

INGREDIENTS:

Maple-Glazed Nuts ingredients:
- 2 cups almonds
- 2 cups walnuts
- $1/2$ cup real maple syrup

Salad ingredients:
- 2 beets, peeled and chopped
- 1 tablespoon extra-virgin olive oil
- sea salt and freshly-ground pepper, to taste
- 6 cups mixed salad greens
- 2 carrots, peeled and shredded
- 1 red bell pepper, diced
- 2 tablespoons hemp hearts
- 2 tablespoons pumpkin seeds
- $1/4$ cup dried cranberries
- $1/2$ cup maple-glazed nuts (from above)

INSTRUCTIONS:

1. To make the topping, heat a dry skillet over medium-high heat, then add in the almonds and walnuts. Pour in the maple syrup and stir to coat the nuts, watching carefully, as nuts can burn quickly. Keep stirring the nuts until the syrup caramelizes and the nuts become sticky.

2. Remove from heat and pour onto a parchment-paper-lined baking sheet.

3. Allow the nuts to harden completely, then break into pieces and set aside.

4. To make the salad, preheat the oven to 350°F.

5. Drizzle the beets with olive oil and salt and pepper, and roast in the oven for 25 minutes.

6. In the meantime, place the salad greens in bowl, and mix together with carrots and red pepper.

7. Top with hemp hearts, pumpkin seeds, cranberries, and maple-glazed nuts and drizzle with the *Creamy Balsamic Vinaigrette* (from the *Sweet n' Savoury Dips and Dressings* section).

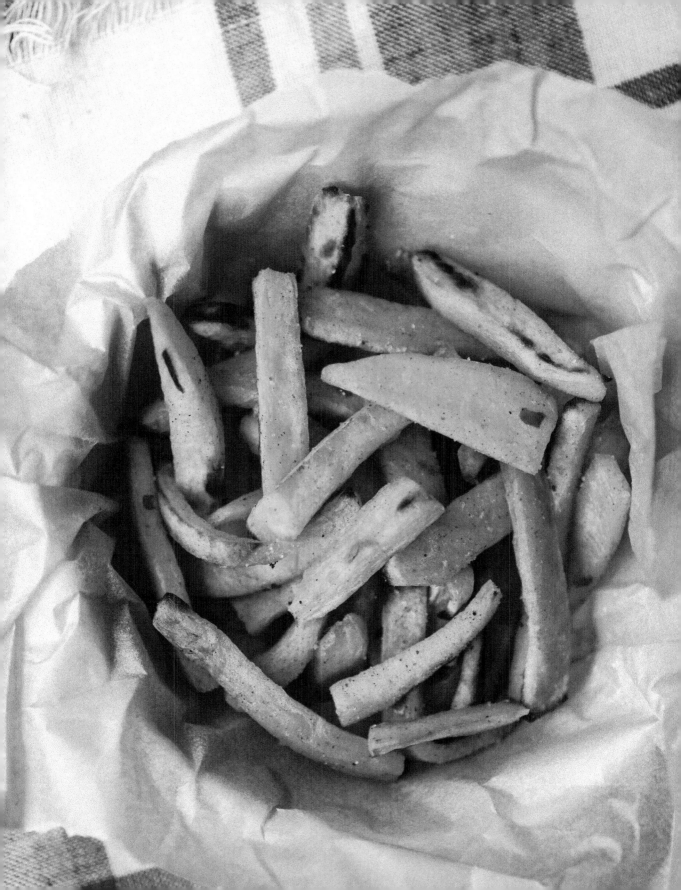

Sweet Potato Fries

Serves 4-6

Salty, sweet and crunchy, these baked sweet potato fries are my family's new favourite side dish. They are a much better choice than traditional fries because they pack a nutritional punch with a day's worth of vitamin A, as well as a good dose of carotenoids and vitamins B and C.

INGREDIENTS:

- 6 medium sweet potatoes, peeled and sliced into long $1/2$ inch thick strips
- 1 teaspoon ground cinnamon
- $1/2$ teaspoon sea salt
- a pinch of cayenne pepper
- 1 $1/2$ tablespoons coconut oil, melted

INSTRUCTIONS:

1. Preheat oven to 400°F.
2. Sprinkle cinnamon, sea salt, and cayenne over sweet potato slices.
3. Pour coconut oil onto potatoes and mix with your hands until well coated.
4. Line two cookie sheets with parchment paper and spread out sweet potatoes on the cookie sheets, trying not to let sweet potatoes overlap.
5. Bake for 25 minutes or until cooked through on the inside and crispy on the outside.
6. Serve immediately.

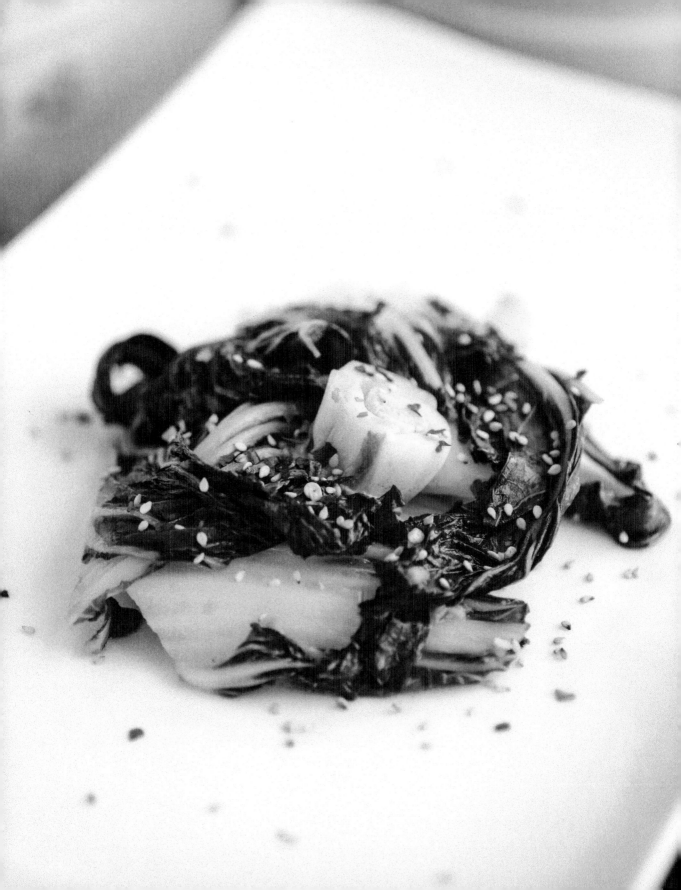

Sautéed Super Greens

Serves 2-4

An excellent source of vitamins A, C, and K, these super-delicious super-greens are the perfect side dish. They can be served with chicken, fish, or burgers, or added on top of a vegan or vegetarian rice or quinoa bowl.

INGREDIENTS:

- 1 tablespoon coconut oil
- 6 cups mixed greens like swiss chard, beet greens, kale, or spinach
- $1/4$ teaspoon each of dried garlic powder, onion powder, parsley, basil, marjoram, rosemary, and thyme
- $1/4$ cup chicken or vegetable broth
- $1/2$ teaspoon sea salt
- optional: 1 tablespoon sesame seeds

INSTRUCTIONS:

1. Heat coconut oil over medium heat. Add greens and spices and sauté for a minute. Add in chicken stock and turn heat to high.

2. Continue to stir, allowing chicken stock to evaporate completely.

3. Sprinkle with sea salt and sesame seeds, if using, and serve.

TIP:
Leafy greens are the most nutrient-rich foods on the planet. For optimal health and to protect yourself from environmental toxins, consume at least 2–3 servings each day. Sneak them into smoothies, soups, meatballs, pastas, stews, stir-frys, sandwiches, dips, dressings, and even desserts.

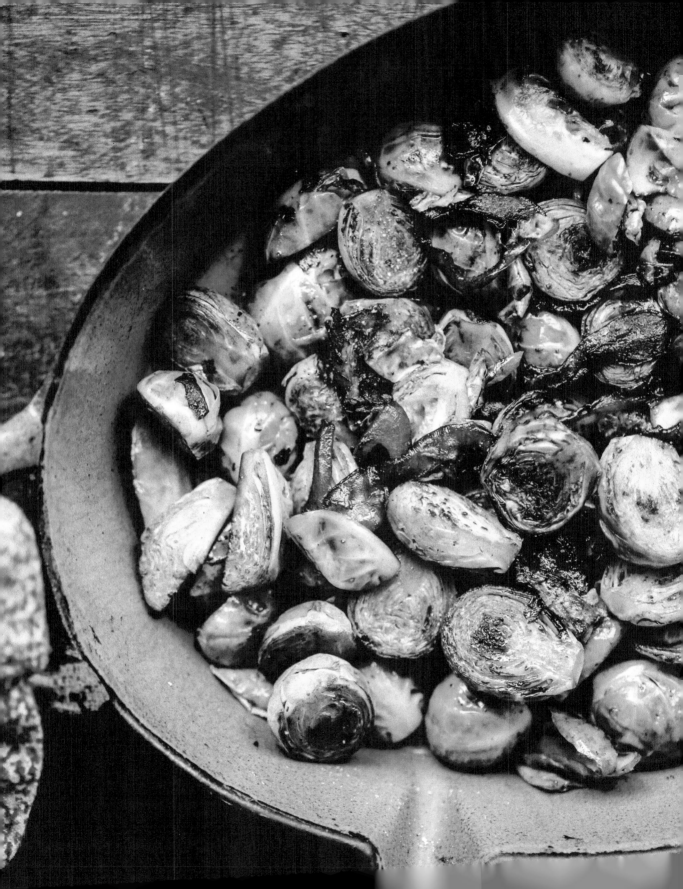

Pan-Roasted Brussels Sprouts

Serves 2-4

Brussels sprouts are a good source of fibre, protein, iron, potassium, folate, and vitamin C. Pan-frying these sprouts with balsamic vinegar caramelizes them beautifully and really brings out their flavour.

INGREDIENTS:

- 1 tablespoon coconut oil or ghee
- 2 cups Brussels sprouts, halved, with ends trimmed
- $1/4$ cup red onion, peeled and chopped
- 1 tablespoon Herbamare
- $1/4$ cup balsamic vinegar

INSTRUCTIONS:

1. In a medium saucepan, heat coconut oil or ghee over medium heat.
2. Add the Brussels sprouts and red onion to the pan and sauté for 2-3 minutes.
3. Add in the Herbamare and vinegar and turn the heat to high, allowing the vinegar to evaporate.
4. Remove from heat and serve.

> TIP: 🍴
>
> Herbamare is an organic seasoning salt which can be found in most local grocery stores. I usually pick mine up at Costco because they carry it in the larger 500 gram version. It's a blend of celery, leek, watercress, onions, chives, parsley, lovage, garlic, basil, marjoram, rosemary, thyme, and kelp, which are all organically grown. I always keep it on hand because it makes pretty much any food taste great.

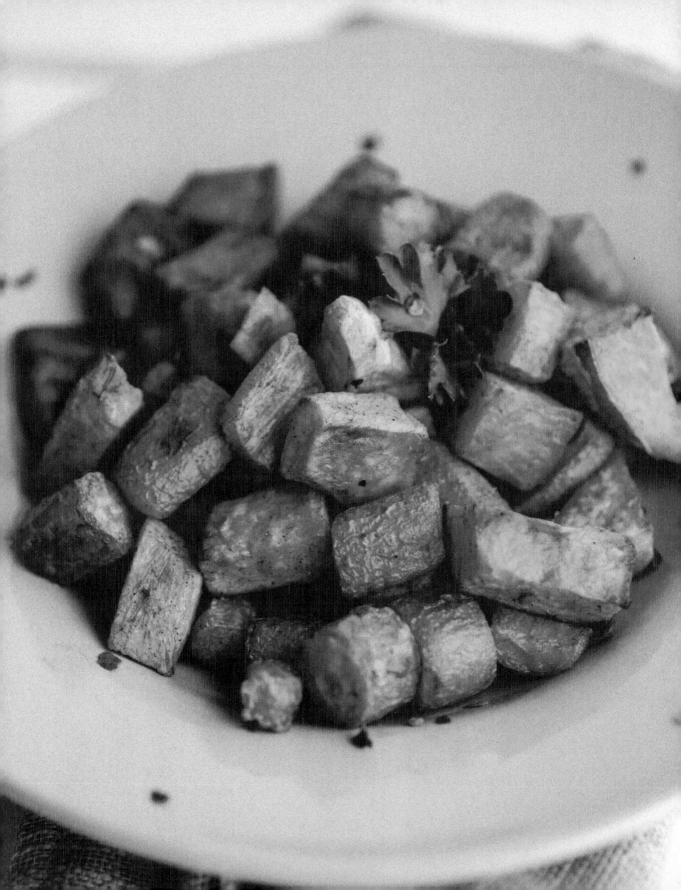

Roasted Carrots and Sweet Potatoes

Serves 4-6

There are few things more comforting than roasted root vegetables, but they also risk being a bit boring if left to their own devices. The trick for turning them from drab to fab is simply to toss them in coconut oil and season them with some fragrant spices.

INGREDIENTS:

- 3 sweet potatoes, peeled and cubed
- 5 heirloom carrots, peeled and chopped into large pieces
- 2 tablespoons coconut oil, melted
- $^1/_2$ teaspoon ground cumin
- $^1/_2$ teaspoon ground cinnamon
- $^1/_4$ teaspoon sea salt
- freshly-ground black pepper, to taste

INSTRUCTIONS:

1. Preheat oven to 400°F.
2. Place potatoes and carrots in a large bowl. Toss in coconut oil, and then sprinkle with remaining ingredients.
3. Spread onto a roasting pan and bake for 30 minutes.
4. Remove from the oven and let cool slightly before serving.

TIP:
Try subbing in other varieties of root vegetables next time you make this dish. You can try beets, parsnips, turnips, yams, or red onions, to name a few. Simply season with some sea salt and freshly ground pepper, or try out some new spice combinations to suit your own palate!

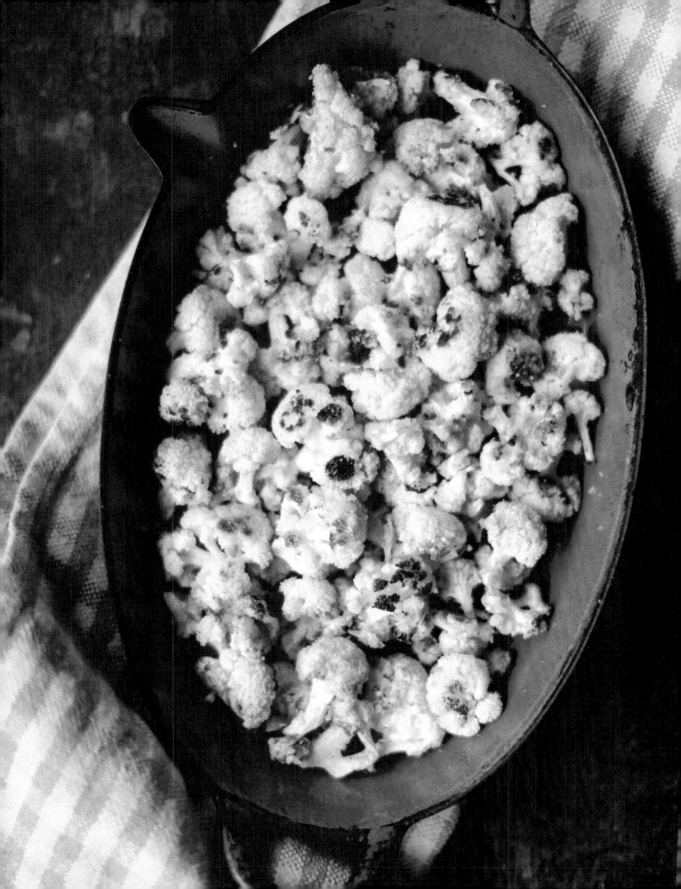

Cauliflower Popcorn

Serves 4-6

This is my absolute favourite way to eat cauliflower. Cauliflower "popcorn" is the perfect snack when you feel like reaching for nutritionally void chips or microwave popcorn, because it satisfies salty and crunchy cravings, but it also works as a savoury side dish. This cauliflower is cheesy and crunchy and a little bit sweet, and the combination of flavours is just divine.

INGREDIENTS:

- 1 head cauliflower, broken into florets
- 2 tablespoons coconut oil, melted
- $^1/_4$ cup nutritional yeast
- 2 tablespoons almond meal
- $^1/_2$ teaspoon sea salt
- freshly-ground black pepper, to taste

INSTRUCTIONS:

1. Preheat oven to 375°F.
2. Place cauliflower in a medium-sized bowl. Pour in the coconut oil and then sprinkle with remaining ingredients, mixing until evenly coated.
3. Spread out in a roasting pan and bake for 20 minutes. Remove from oven and serve.

> **TIP:**
>
> Most vegetables taste great when tossed in coconut oil, seasoned, and roasted in the oven. I usually bake my veggies (try a combo of cauliflower florets, broccoli spears, and red onion) at 400°F for 10 minutes, then I add some chopped kale (massaged in coconut oil and sprinkled with sea salt) on top and roast it all for another 10 minutes. Bingo - it's done!

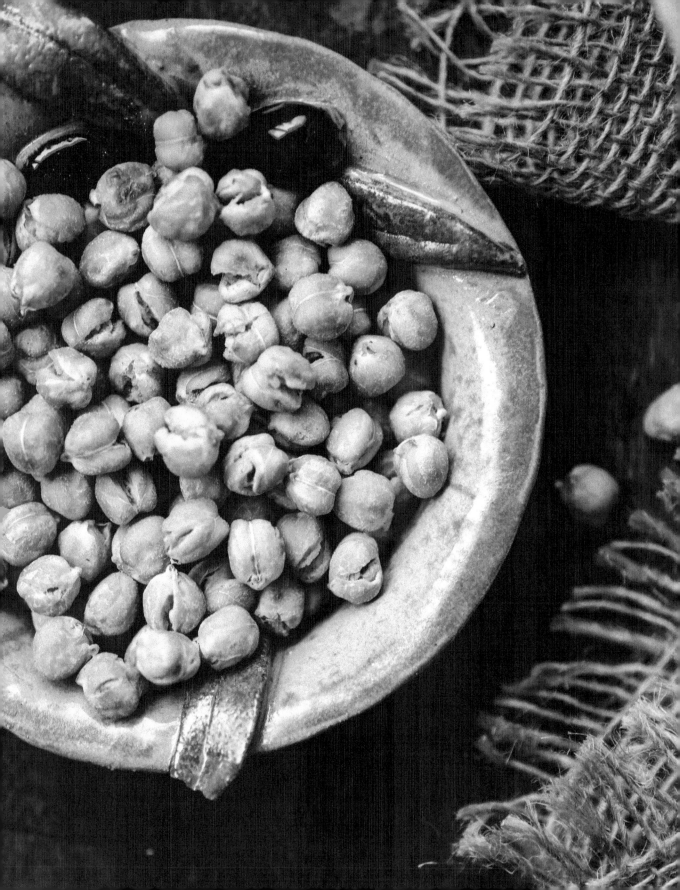

Roasted Chickpeas, two ways

Makes 1 1/2 cups

Roasted chickpeas are one of my favourite salad and soup toppers ever! They are also a great snack and can be served as a side as well. So simple to make, crunchy, high in protein, and incredibly satisfying, you will want to keep a container of these on hand at all times.

INGREDIENTS:

- 1 (14-ounce) can chickpeas, drained, rinsed and patted dry
- 1–1 1/2 tablespoons coconut oil, melted
- 1 teaspoon dried oregano
- 1 teaspoon chili powder
- 1 teaspoon ground cumin
- ¼ teaspoon sea salt
- freshly-ground pepper, to taste

OR

- 1 (14-ounce) can chickpeas, drained, rinsed and patted dry
- 1–1 1/2 tablespoons coconut oil, melted
- 1 tablespoon curry powder
- 1/4 teaspoon sea salt
- freshly-ground pepper, to taste

INSTRUCTIONS:

1. Preheat oven to 400°F. Place the oven rack in the middle of the oven.

2. Place chickpeas in a medium-sized bowl, and drizzle with melted coconut oil, sea salt, and spices, and mix until well coated.

3. Place chickpeas on a baking sheet, spread them out evenly, and bake for 35-40 minutes or until crisp, stirring every 10 minutes.

4. Remove from oven when done and set aside to cool slightly, then serve.

TIP:
To save time, you can pan-fry these in coconut oil instead of roasting them. Simply add the chickpeas, coconut oil, and spices to a hot pan and pan-fry them over medium-high heat for about 10 minutes. Make sure to stir constantly so the chickpeas don't burn.

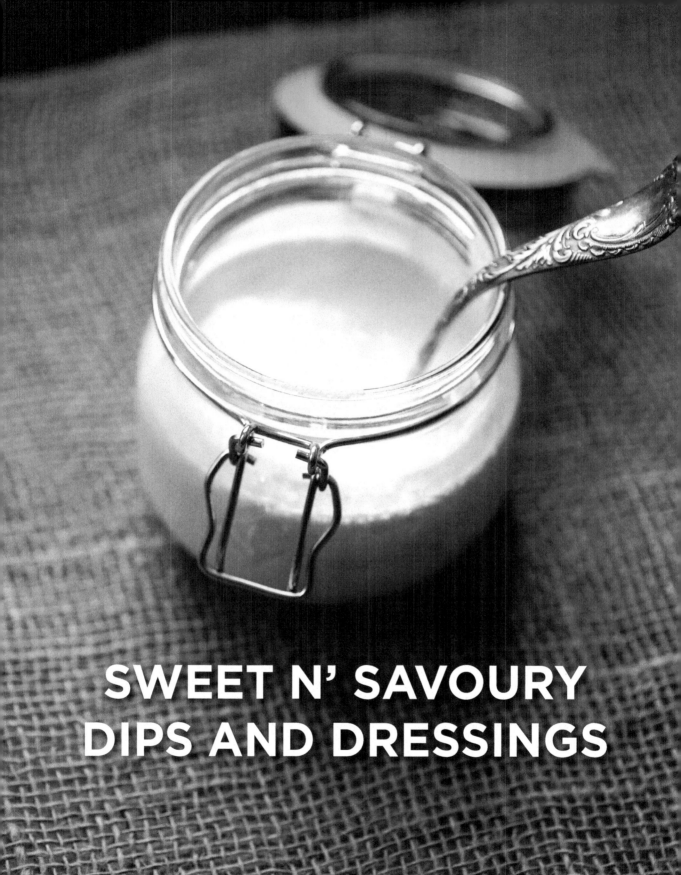

SWEET N' SAVOURY
DIPS AND DRESSINGS

Apple-Cider Vinaigrette

Makes 2 cups

This apple-cider vinaigrette captures the essence of fall. Incredibly alkalizing and full of raw enzymes and probiotics, it's great for aiding with the digestive process as well. Pour it over some greens, drizzle it onto a quinoa or rice bowl, or brush it onto some pork chops before grilling.

INGREDIENTS:

- $1/4$ cup freshly-squeezed lemon juice
- $1/4$ cup extra-virgin olive oil
- $1/8$ cup raw apple cider vinegar
- 1 tablespoon dijon mustard
- 1 tablespoon maple syrup
- 1–2 cloves garlic, crushed
- $1/2$ teaspoon sea salt
- $1/4$ teaspoon pepper
- a pinch of dried oregano

INSTRUCTIONS:

1. Add all ingredients to a food processor and blend until smooth.
2. Store in the fridge in an air-tight, glass container for up to a week.

NOTE:

This recipe was created by Culinary Nutrition Expert and co-owner of Bliss B4 Laundry retreats, Gabriela Flores, and is being printed with her permission. To learn more about these amazing women's wellness retreats, check out their website www.blissb4laundry.com.

Blueberry Vinaigrette

Makes 2 cups

This is probably my favourite dressing of all time. It is light, sweet, and tangy, and versatile enough to go well with almost any salad, plus it is packed with antioxidants and vitamin C, making it the perfect choice for when your immune system needs a boost.

INGREDIENTS:

- 1 cup blueberries
- $^1/_4$ cup freshly-squeezed lemon juice
- $^1/_4$ cup balsamic vinegar
- $^1/_2$ cup grapeseed or avocado oil
- 1 tablespoon real maple syrup
- 1 $^1/_2$ teaspoons Dijon mustard
- $^1/_4$ teaspoon sea salt

INSTRUCTIONS:

1. Add all ingredients to a food processor and mix together until vinaigrette thickens and no blueberry pieces remain.

2. Store in the fridge in an air-tight, glass container for up to a week.

TIP:

Cup per cup, wild blueberries have twice as much antioxidant power as cultivated varieties, plus they are normally grown without any pesticides because they are naturally more resistant to pests and insects.

Spicy Tahini Dressing

Makes 2 cups

This dressing is deliciously smooth and creamy and goes well with pretty much any meal. I particularly like it on Buddha Bowls! The tahini is high in calcium and protein so you stay satisfied for longer, and the parsley and lemon juice are great for boosting your immune system and assisting in detoxification.

INGREDIENTS:

- $1/4$ cup tahini
- $1/4$ cup freshly-squeezed lemon juice
- $3/4$ cup water
- 2 tablespoons fresh parsley
- $1/2$ teaspoon sea salt
- $1/4$ teaspoon cayene or red pepper flakes

INSTRUCTIONS:

1. To make dressing, add all ingredients to a food processor and blend until smooth.

2. Store in the fridge in an air-tight, glass container for up to a week.

NOTE:

This recipe was created by Culinary Nutrition Expert and co-owner of Bliss B4 Laundry retreats, Gabriela Flores and is being shared with her permission. Gabriela is a chef extraordinaire and regularly cooks for 75 people in one sitting!

Maple Dijon Dressing

Makes 1 ¹/₄ cups

The combination of Dijon mustard and maple syrup create a sweet and tangy sensation that will delight your taste buds. This versatile dressing can be drizzled over salad or roasted vegetables or be used as a marinade for chicken or pork.

INGREDIENTS:

- ¹/₄ cup extra-virgin olive oil
- ¹/₂ cup apple cider vinegar
- ¹/₄ cup Dijon mustard
- 2 tablespoons real maple syrup
- a pinch of sea salt
- a pinch of cayenne

INSTRUCTIONS:

1. To make dressing, whisk together all ingredients in a small bowl until well combined, or alternatively, add all ingredients to a food processor and blend until smooth.

2. Dressing can be stored in the fridge in an air-tight, glass container for up to a week.

TIP:

Drinking raw apple cider vinegar (ACV) in water can help to naturally improve your digestion. Just add a tablespoon of ACV to a large glass of water 15 minutes before a meal to stimulate your digestive juices and facilitate the breakdown of food. My favourite brand is Bragg Organic Apple Cider Vinegar. Find it in your local health food store.

Avocado Dressing

Makes 1 ¹/₂ cups

This gorgeous green dressing will make your world go round! Avocado is so nutrient dense, it's often referred to as a superfood. Incredibly high in fibre, healthy fats, B vitamins, vitamin K, vitamin C, and potassium, plus a host of many other trace minerals, avocados really deliver bang for your buck!

INGREDIENTS:

- 1 avocado, peeled and pitted
- ¹/₂ medium onion, peeled and quartered
- 1 green pepper, seeded and quartered
- 2 cloves garlic, peeled
- 1 cup fresh cilantro leaves
- ¹/₂ cup fresh parsely leaves
- 1 tablespoon real maple syrup
- ¹/₂ cup white vinegar
- 2 tablespoons freshly-squeezed lemon or lime juice
- 1 cup water
- sea salt and freshly-ground pepper, to taste

INSTRUCTIONS:

1. To make dressing, add all ingredients to a food processor and blend until smooth.
2. Store in the fridge in an air-tight, glass container for up to a week.

> **NOTE:**
> This recipe was created by Culinary Nutrition Expert and co-owner of Bliss B4 Laundry retreats, Gabriela Flores, and is being shared with her permission.

> **TIP:**
> Avocados are also called alligator pears due to their pear-like shape and green, bumpy skin.

Creamy Balsamic Vinaigrette

Makes 1 ¹/₂ cups

This creamy dressing is so yummy and so simple to make that you may never buy store-bought dressing again. It pairs beautifully with spring greens topped with fresh or dried berries and oven-roasted nuts.

INGREDIENTS:

- ¹/₂ cup plus 1 tablespoon balsamic vinegar
- 3 tablespoons Dijon mustard
- 1 tablespoon raw honey
- ³/₄ cup extra-virgin olive oil
- sea salt and freshly-ground pepper, to taste

INSTRUCTIONS:

1. Whisk together the vinegar, mustard, and honey in a medium-sized bowl.
2. Slowly pour in olive oil in a steady stream, whisking as you go.
3. Season with salt and pepper to taste.
4. Store in the fridge in an air-tight, glass container for up to a week.

Balsamic Honey-Maple Dressing

Makes 1 cup

A good balsamic dressing should be a staple in every household. I love this one because it can be whipped up in less than five minutes with only five ingredients. It is both sweet and tangy and pairs well with any green salad. It also works well as marinade for chicken or pork.

INGREDIENTS:

- $^1/_4$ cup Dijon mustard
- $^1/_4$ cup extra-virgin olive oil
- $^1/_4$ cup balsamic vinegar
- 2 tablespoons raw honey
- 2 tablespoons real maple syrup

INSTRUCTIONS:

1. To make dressing, whisk the first three ingredients together in a small bowl until the mixture thickens, then whisk in the honey and maple syrup. Alternatively, you can add all ingredients to a food processor and blend until smooth.

2. Store in the fridge in an air-tight, glass container for up to a week.

Creamy Miso Dressing

Makes 2 cups

Creamy and dreamy with none of the guilt – what more could you want from a dressing? Well, this one over-delivers. Anti-viral, anti-bacterial and anti-inflammatory, high in protein and healthy fat, this is a dressing you will make over and over again.

INGREDIENTS:

- $^3/_4$ cup firm organic tofu
- 2 cloves of garlic, peeled and crushed
- $^1/_4$ cup tahini
- 2 teaspoons miso paste
- 2 tablespoons raw apple cider vinegar
- 1 tablespoon raw honey
- 2 tablespoons freshly-squeezed lemon juice
- 2 teaspoons nutritional yeast
- 3 tablespoons extra-virgin olive oil
- 2 teaspoons tamari
- $^1/_2$ teaspoon sea salt
- $^1/_2$ cup water

INSTRUCTIONS:

1. Add all dressing ingredients to a food processor and blend until smooth.
2. Store in the fridge in an air-tight, glass container for up to a week.

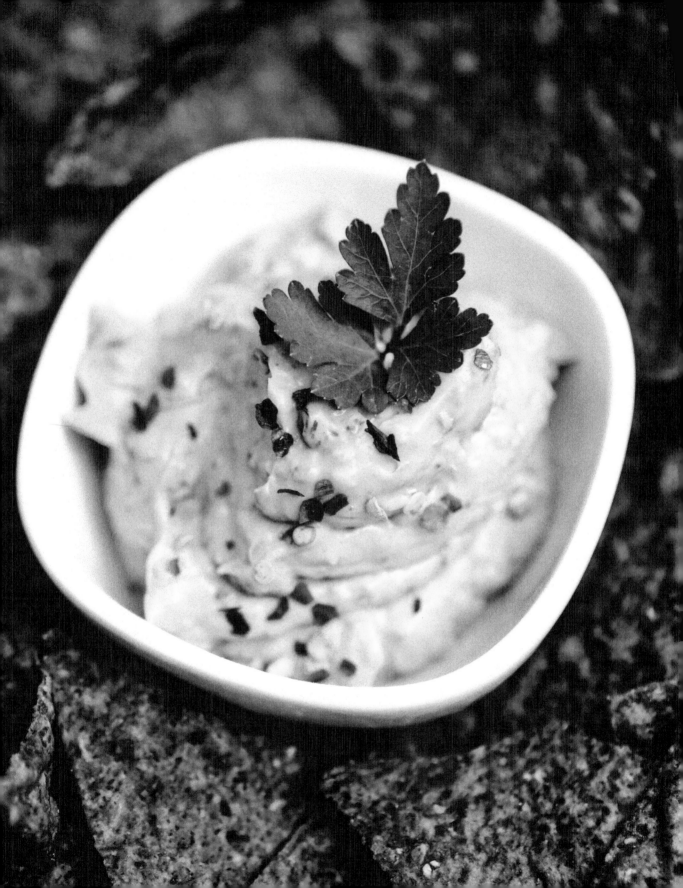

Spinach-Avocado Dip

Serves 6-8

Spinach and avocado are blended together to make this gorgeous, nutrient-packed, superfood dip, which can also be used as a spread for wraps or sandwiches. High in vitamins A, E, and K, and full of fibre, iron, calcium, and phytonutrients, this is a dip you will actually feel good about eating. My kids love it too!

INGREDIENTS:

- 2 avocados, peeled and sliced
- 1 cup organic baby spinach
- $^1/_2$ sweet onion, peeled and chopped
- 2 tablespoons freshly-squeezed lime juice
- $^1/_2$ teaspoon sea salt
- a pinch of cayenne

INSTRUCTIONS:

1. Blend everything together in a food processor until smooth.
2. Serve with crackers, on top of bread, or as a dip for veggie sticks.
3. Store in the fridge in an air-tight, glass container for 3–5 days.

TIP:
If you're serving this to the kids, you may want to omit the cayenne.

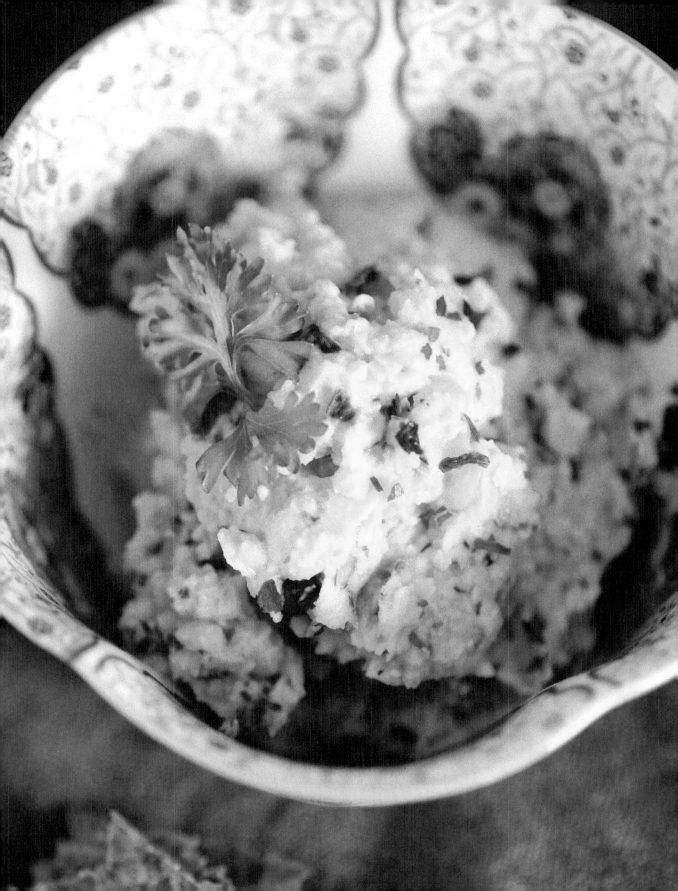

Spicy Hummus

Serves 6–8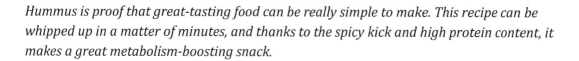

Hummus is proof that great-tasting food can be really simple to make. This recipe can be whipped up in a matter of minutes, and thanks to the spicy kick and high protein content, it makes a great metabolism-boosting snack.

INGREDIENTS:

- 1 (14-ounce) can chickpeas, drained and rinsed
- $^1/_4$ cup freshly-squeezed lemon juice
- $^1/_2$ cup water
- $^1/_4$ cup tahini
- 2 tablespoon extra-virgin olive oil
- 1 clove garlic, peeled and crushed
- 1 teaspoon sea salt
- 1 teaspoon chili powder
- 1 teasoon dried oregano
- 1 teaspoon ground cumin

INSTRUCTIONS:

1. Blend everything together in a food processor until smooth.
2. Store in the fridge in an air-tight, glass container for 3–5 days.

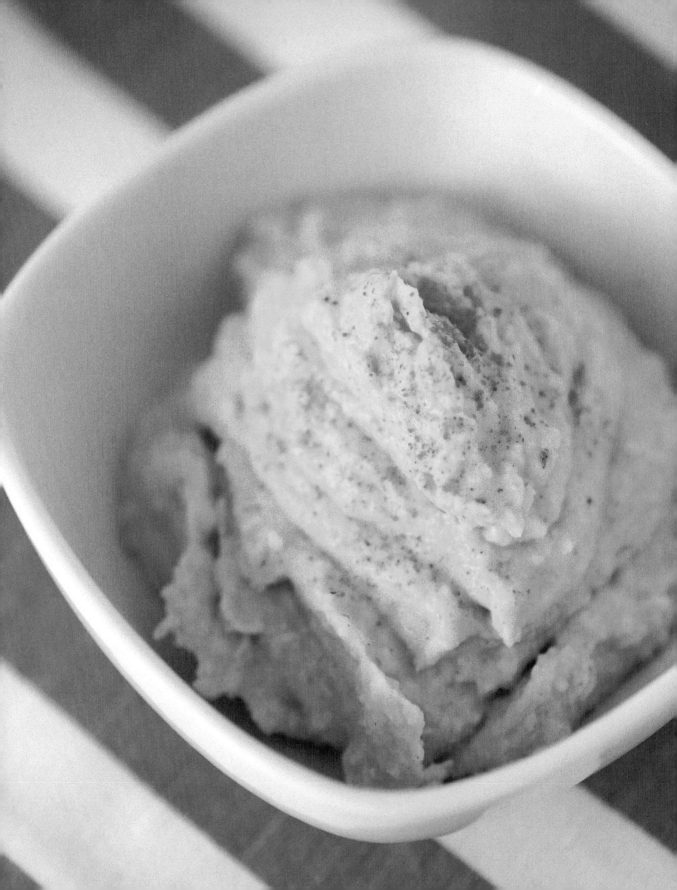

Classic Hummus

Makes 2 cups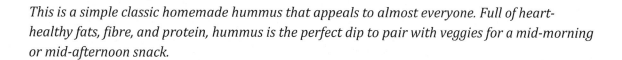

This is a simple classic homemade hummus that appeals to almost everyone. Full of heart-healthy fats, fibre, and protein, hummus is the perfect dip to pair with veggies for a mid-morning or mid-afternoon snack.

INGREDIENTS:

- 2 (14-ounce) cans chickpeas
- $1/2$ cup liquid reserved liquid from chickpeas
- juice from ½ a lemon
- $1/2$ cup tahini
- 2 garlic cloves, peeled and minced
- 2 teaspoons sea salt
- 2 teaspoons ground cumin
- $1/2$–1 teaspoon dried paprika
- 1 tablespoon extra-virgin olive oil

INSTRUCTIONS:

1. Drain and rinse chickpeas, retaining $1/2$ cup of the liquid from one can.
2. Blend together rinsed chickpeas with reserved liquid in a food processor until smooth.
3. Add remaining ingredients, and blend until smooth.
4. Store in the fridge in an air-tight, glass container for 3–5 days.

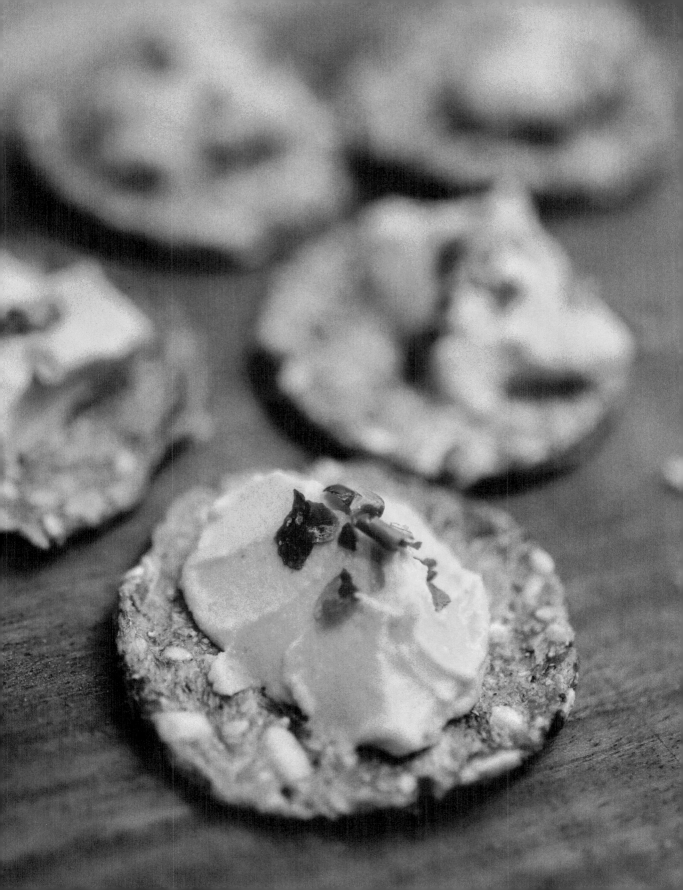

Roasted Carrot Hummus

Serves 8

Roasted carrots add a unique twist to traditional hummus and are an excellent source of beta-carotene, which is great for preventing cancer, slowing down aging, and improving vision. The roasted carrots provide a slightly sweet flavour to the hummus, which kids love.

INGREDIENTS:

- 5 carrots, halved lengthwise, then sliced
- 1–2 tablespoons extra-virgin olive oil
- 1 teaspoon sea salt
- 1 small garlic clove, peeled and crushed
- 2 tablespoons tahini
- 1 (14-ounce) can chickpeas, drained and rinsed
- $1/4$ cup water
- juice of 1 lemon
- $1/2$–1 teaspoon ground cumin
- $1/4$ teaspoon dried paprika
- 1 teaspoon sea salt
- fresh cilantro for garnish

INSTRUCTIONS:

1. Preheat oven to 350°F.
2. Place carrots on a baking sheet, drizzle with olive oil, and sprinkle with sea salt.
3. Roast for 30 minutes, then remove from oven and let cool.
4. In the meantime, mix together remaining ingredients in a food processor until well-blended.
5. Once carrots have cooled enough to handle, add to food processor, and process until smooth, adding a bit more water if necessary.
6. Garnish with some cilantro and serve with veggies or gluten-free crackers.
7. Store leftovers in the fridge in an air-tight, glass container for 3–5 days.

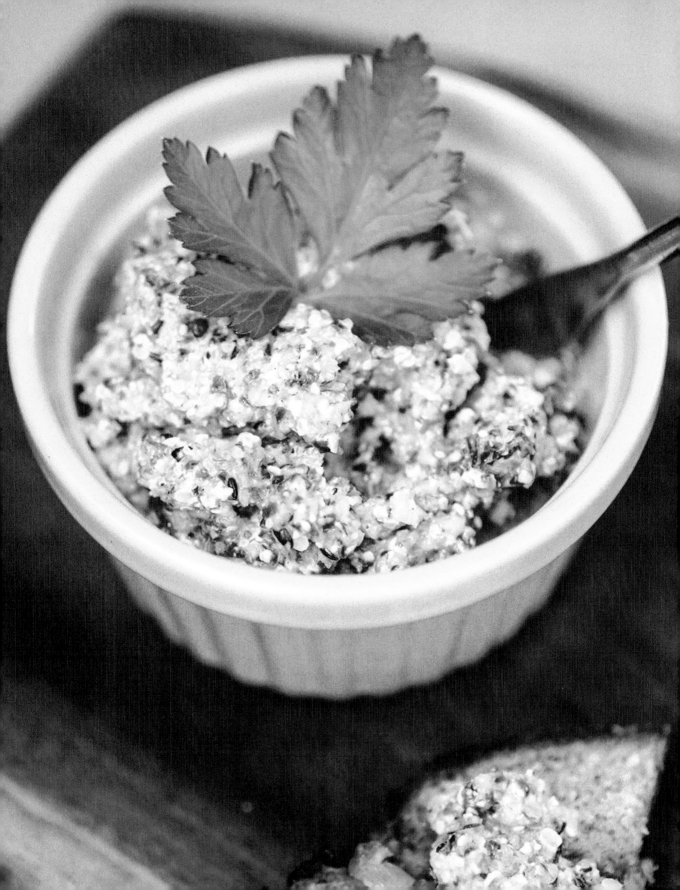

Zucchini-Hemp Hummus

Serves 6–8

Zucchinis are incredibly versatile and, when combined with hemp hearts, act as a creamy base for this wonderful dip. Of course, I had to sneak in some spinach for extra greens and a bit of cilantro for a slightly spicy kick.

INGREDIENTS:

- juice of $1/2$ lemon
- 1 small garlic clove, peeled and crushed
- 2 tablespoons extra-virgin olive oil
- 1 medium or large zucchini, chopped
- 1 cup baby spinach, packed
- $1/4$ cup fresh cilantro
- $1/2$ cup hemp hearts
- 1 teaspoon sea salt
- a pinch of cayenne

INSTRUCTIONS:

1. Blend everything together in a high-powered food processor until smooth.
2. Store in the fridge in an air-tight, glass container for 3–5 days.

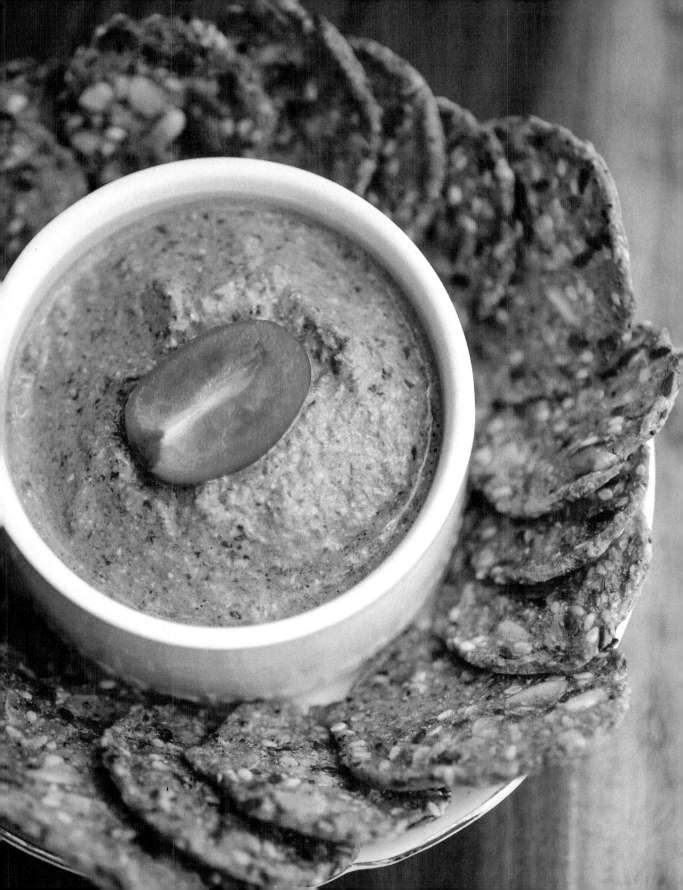

Spinach-Hempseed Pesto

Serves 6–8

Popeye would have been envious of this protein-packed, iron-rich, detoxifying, alkalizing, nutrient-dense and delicious dip! Feel great and look even better after you have dolloped this dip onto crackers, veggies, eggs, spiralized zucchini noodles, or gluten-free pasta. Try it with the Vegan Falafel or the Nutty Bean Burgers from the Entreés section.

INGREDIENTS:

- 2 cups fresh basil leaves
- 2 cups baby spinach
- $^1/_3$ cup hemp hearts
- 2 tablespoons flaxseed oil
- 3 tablespoons nutritional yeast
- juice of $^1/_2$ lemon (about 2 tablespoons)
- 1 teaspoon garlic powder
- $^1/_2$ teaspoon sea salt
- 2–3 tablespoons water, to reach desired consistency

INSTRUCTIONS:

1. Add all ingredients to a food processor and blend until smooth.
2. Store in the fridge in an air-tight, glass container for 3–5 days.

NOTE:

This lovely pesto recipe was slightly adapted from the *Basil-Spinach Pesto* recipe by McKel Hill[46] on www.nutritionstripped.com, which is one of my favourite healthy-cooking websites ever.

TIP:

If you are vegan or just trying to give up dairy, nutritional yeast is soon to become your new BFF. Incredibly high in B vitamins, protein, fibre, selenium and chromium, this inactive yeast tastes like cheese! Yes, you heard it right! Sprinkle it on top of pasta to mimic parmesan cheese, blend it with cashews and lemon juice for a vegan cream cheese, or pair it with butternut squash, Dijon mustard, coconut milk and lemon juice for a faux Mac n' Cheese that may even fool the kids! My favourite brand is Bragg Nutritional Yeast Seasoning which you can find at your local health food store.

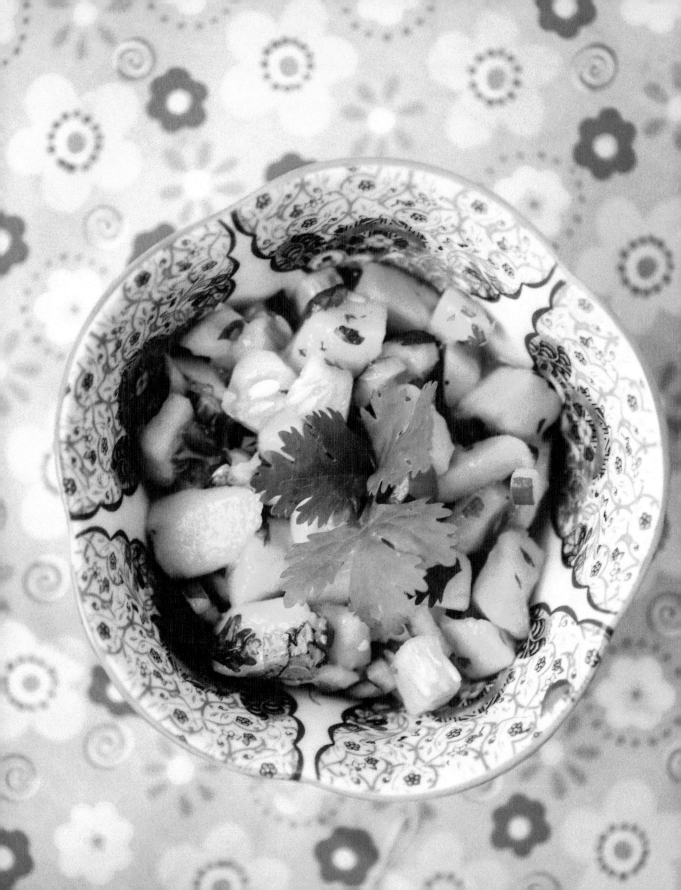

Mango Salsa

Makes 2 cups

This gorgeous salsa is light and refreshing, making it a perfect side dish for a hot summer's day. The mangos provide vitamins A, C, and folate, the cilantro has great antibacterial properties and assists with detoxification, and the cucumbers help cool the body and fight inflammation.

INGREDIENTS:

- 1 ripe mango, finely diced
- $^1/_2$ English cucumber, peeled and seeded, finely diced
- $^1/_2$ medium red onion, peeled and finely diced
- a handful of fresh cilantro (approximately $^1/_4$ cup), finely chopped
- 1–2 limes, juiced
- optional: 1 small jalapeno, seeded and finely diced
- optional: garnish with chopped fresh green onions

INSTRUCTIONS:

1. To make salsa, mix together all ingredients in a small bowl.
2. Serve salsa on its own, as a side, or pair it with the *Fish Tacos* (from the *Entrées section*).
3. Salsa can be stored in the fridge in an air-tight, glass container for up to 2–3 days.

NOTE:

This recipe was created by my good friend and dietician, Ariadne Legendre, and is being printed with her permission.

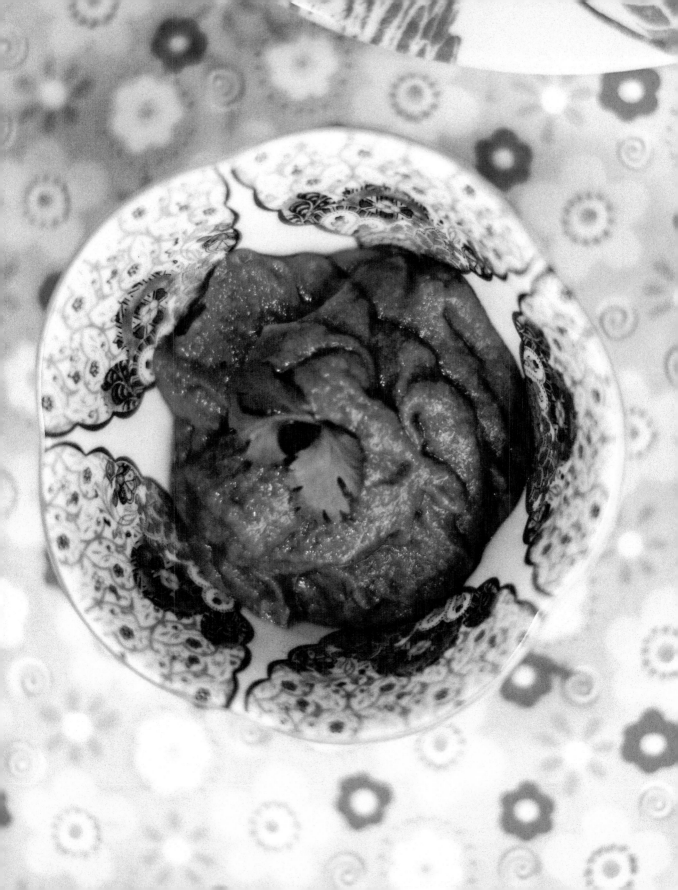

Chipotle Dipping Sauce

Makes 1 ¹/₂ cups

Cool, creamy and spicy, this sauce is incredibly versatile and can be paired with pretty much any food. Try it with the Fish Tacos (from the Entrées section), the Sweet Potato Fries (from the Soups, Salads and Sides section), or drizzled over fresh vegetables, burgers or grilled chicken.

INGREDIENTS:

- 1 cup full-fat coconut milk
- 5 sundried tomatoes (dry, not in oil)
- ¹/₃ cup cashews
- 1–1 ¹/₂ tablespoons tamari sauce
- 1 chipotle pepper or ¹/₂ jalapeno pepper

INSTRUCTIONS:

1. Place all ingredients in a blender and mix until smooth.

2. If the sauce seems too thick, add a bit of water, one teaspoon at a time, until you reach the desired consistency.

3. Store in the fridge in an air-tight, glass container for 2–3 days.

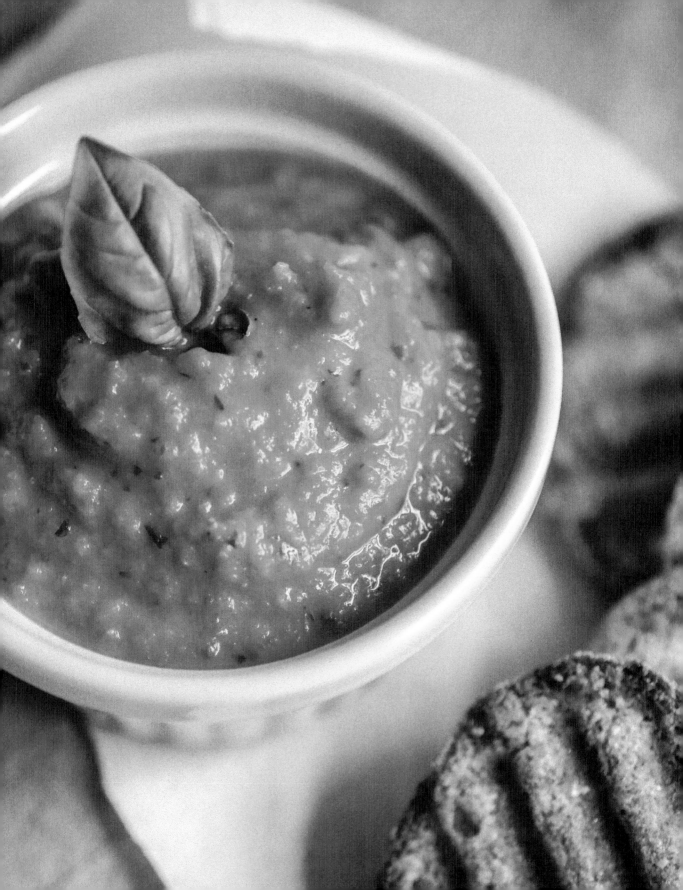

Roasted-Red-Pepper Dipping Sauce

Serves 10-12

Roasted red pepper gives this sauce a slightly sweet taste and gorgeous colour, plus they are incredibly high in vitamin C and beta carotene, which are potent immune boosters. Serve this as a dipping sauce for meatballs or veggies, or as a pizza or pasta sauce.

INGREDIENTS:

- 2 red bell peppers, halved and seeded
- $1/4$ cup extra-virgin olive oil
- $1/2$ cup white onion, peeled and chopped
- 4 cups cherry tomatoes, chopped
- 2 large carrots, peeled and shredded
- 4 cloves garlic, peeled and crushed
- 1 can organic tomato paste
- 1 cup fresh basil, chopped
- $1/4$ cup fresh flat leaf parsley, chopped
- 2 teaspoons dried oregano
- 1 teaspoon dried thyme
- $1/2$ teaspoon freshly-ground black pepper
- 2 tablespoons real maple syrup
- 2 teaspoons sea salt

INSTRUCTIONS:

1. Preheat oven to 400°F.

2. Place the peppers, skin-side-up, on a baking sheet near the top of the oven, and roast for 20–30 minutes, until the skin starts to blacken.

3. Remove the peppers from the oven and let cool, then peel off the skin, and chop the peppers into small pieces.

4. Heat the olive oil in a skillet, and then add onions and sauté until translucent.

5. Add the chopped tomatoes, carrots, roasted red peppers, garlic, and tomato paste, and stir for a few minutes, allowing the flavours of the vegetables to blend together.

6. Add in basil, parsley, oregano, thyme, pepper, maple syrup, and sea salt, and simmer on low for about 20 minutes or until the tomatoes are cooked and the sauce thickens.

7. Remove from heat and allow to cool slightly. Once cool enough to handle, pour into a food processor and blend until smooth, about 3–4 minutes, allowing some texture to remain.

8. Dipping sauce can be served warm or cold.

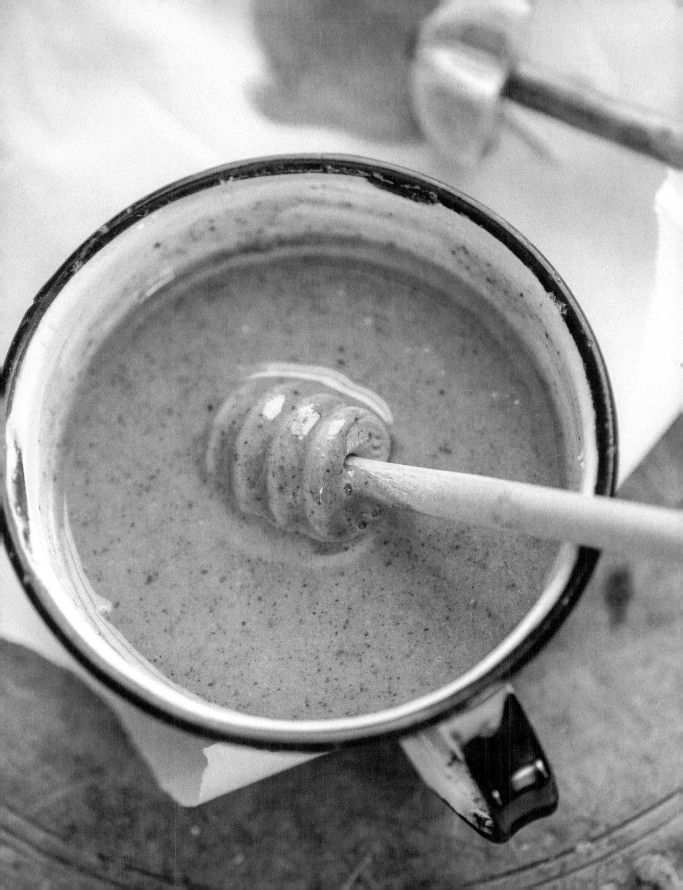

Raw Vegan Caramel Sauce

Serves 10-12

This raw caramel sauce is the perfect alternative for traditional caramel sauce, which is full of dairy and sugar and requires a long cooking time. Luckily, this version is just as delicious and gooey as the original. Serve it drizzled over oatmeal or apple slices, or with homemade banana ice cream.

INGREDIENTS:

- 2 pitted dates, soaked 1-2 hours
- 3 tablespoons coconut oil
- $^1/_4$ cup almond butter
- $^1/_2$ cup real maple syrup
- 1 tablespoon full-fat coconut milk
- 1 teaspoon pure vanilla extract
- $^1/_4$ teaspoon sea salt

INSTRUCTIONS:

1. Blend all ingredients together in a food processor until smooth.

2. Serve immediately or store in the fridge in an air-tight, glass container for up to a week.

TIP:

If you are not using the caramel sauce immediately, it will need to be re-heated prior to use as the coconut oil will harden in the fridge.

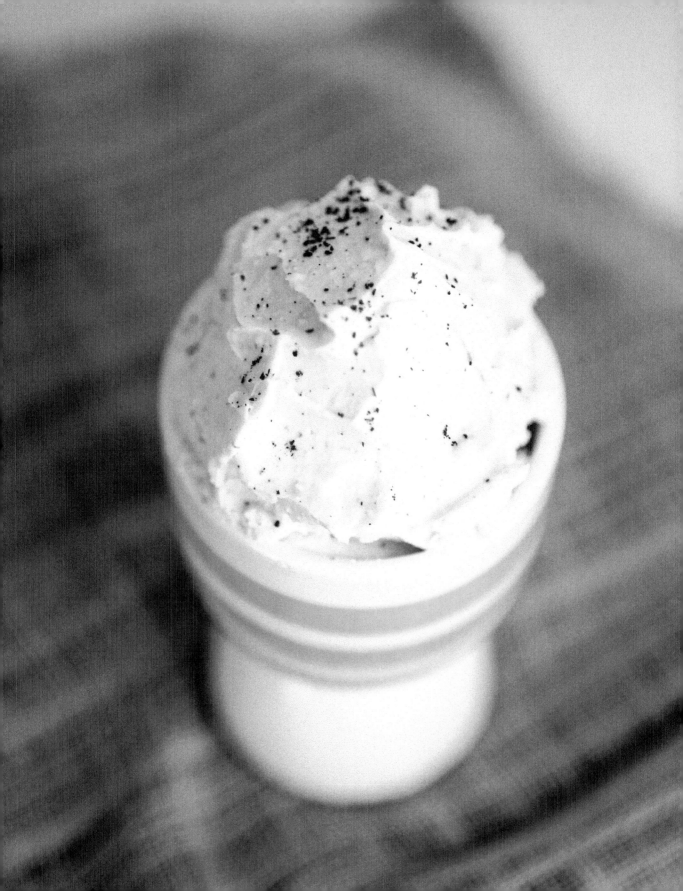

Coconut Whipped Cream

Serves 12–14

I don't know who came up with the idea of Coconut Whipped Cream, but it's the best thing that has been invented in a long time. It completes pretty much any dessert, because it's wonderfully smooth and creamy and yet not too sweet. I will warn you that it's a bit addictive, but your secret is safe with me if you decide to eat it by the spoonful.

INGREDIENTS:

- 1 can of full-fat coconut milk, chilled in the fridge overnight
- seeds of 1 vanilla bean
- 2–3 teaspoons real maple syrup

INSTRUCTIONS:

1. Remove the coconut milk from the fridge, scoop off the thick cream that forms at the top of the can, and place the cream in your stand mixer. Reserve the remaining liquid for smoothies.

2. Using the whisk attachment of your stand mixer, whip the cream until it becomes light and fluffy. Add in the vanilla bean and the maple syrup, and whip for a few more seconds.

3. Use immediately or store in the fridge in an air-tight, glass container for 3–4 days.

TIP:

My favourite brand of full-fat coconut milk for making *Coconut Whipped Cream* is Earth's Choice Organic Coconut Milk. I find that it whips up like a charm and most closely resembles real whipping cream. I like to add a dollop to my morning coffee along with a pinch of cinnamon.

Chocolate-Orange Glaze

Makes 1 cup

A hint of orange makes this simple chocolate glaze stand out from ordinary chocolate sauces. I like to drizzle it over doughnuts, cakes, loaves, or energy balls. I especially recommend it drizzled over the Chocolate-Pumpkin Loaf (from the Desserts and Treats section).

INGREDIENTS:

- 3 tablespoons coconut oil
- 1 cup dairy-free mini chocolate chips
- 2–3 drops orange extract
- a pinch of sea salt

INSTRUCTIONS:

1. To make the glaze, melt the coconut oil and chocolate chips in a saucepan over low-medium heat, stirring constantly so the chocolate doesn't burn.

2. Once melted, remove the saucepan from the heat and stir in the orange extract and salt.

3. Use immediately or store in the fridge in an air-tight, glass container for up to two weeks.

> **TIP:**
> My favourite brand of dairy-free chocolate chips are made by Enjoy Life. They taste just like regular chocolate chips but are made without any of the "top eight" allergens: wheat/gluten, dairy, peanuts, tree nuts, egg, soy, fish and shellfish. All of their products are also made without casein, potato, sesame and sulfites. It's safe to say that I am a huge fan!

Chocolate Sauce

Makes ³/₄ cup

Who would have thought that by mixing together these three healthy ingredients you can create a decadent, delicious and healthful chocolate sauce? High levels of antioxidants, minerals, and energizing fats make this sauce a hit with kids and parents alike. Drizzle atop chocolate desserts or use as a dip for chocolate-covered strawberries.

INGREDIENTS:

- 3 tablespoons coconut oil
- 5 tablespoons raw cacao powder
- 3 tablespoons real maple syrup

INSTRUCTIONS:

1. Melt the coconut oil in a small pot, then turn off the heat, and whisk in the raw cacao and maple syrup till smooth.

2. Use immediately or store in the fridge in an air-tight, glass container for up to two weeks.

> **TIP:**
> If you are not using the chocolate sauce immediately, it will need to be re-heated prior to use as the coconut oil will harden in the fridge.

Cream Cheese Icing

Makes 1 ¹/₂ cups

This cream cheese icing is one of my favourites! It is super easy to make (just make sure to soak your cashews ahead of time) and it tastes just like the real thing. Plus, it's low in sugar, has tons of healthy fats, and a good dose of protein as well. Spread it on cake or just eat it by the spoonful!

INGREDIENTS:

- 1 ¹/₂ cups cashews, soaked overnight
- ¹/₄ cup coconut oil, softened
- ¹/₄ cup real maple syrup
- 2 tablespoons freshly-squeezed lemon juice
- 2 tablespoons pineapple juice
- a pinch of sea salt

INSTRUCTIONS:

1. Add all ingredients to a food processor and mix until completely smooth.

2. Chill in the fridge for about an hour before spreading on cake, cookies or muffins.

3. This icing tastes divine with the *Carrot Cake* (from the *Desserts and Treats* section).

> **TIP:**
> Cashews are great for mimicking a creamy, smooth texture in dairy-free cooking and raw desserts. Just make sure to soak your cashews overnight and rinse them well before using.

Blueberry Chia Seed Jam

Makes 1 ¹/₂ cups

This is a jam you actually want in your fridge! It not only tastes incredible, but because it's low in sugar and high in protein, fibre, antioxidants and healthy fats, it won't spike your blood sugar like most conventional jams will.

INGREDIENTS:

- 2 cups fresh blueberries
- 2 tablespoons freshly-squeezed lemon juice
- ¹/₂ teaspoon lemon rind
- ¹/₄ cup real maple syrup
- 2 ¹/₂ tablespoons chia seeds
- ¹/₂ teaspoon ground cinnamon
- ¹/₄ teaspoon ground cloves

INSTRUCTIONS:

1. Add the blueberries to a medium-sized pot and mash them slightly with a potato masher.

2. Add lemon juice, rind and maple syrup and bring to a boil.

3. Turn down the heat to low-medium and simmer for ten minutes, stirring constantly.

4. Remove from the heat and stir in the chia seeds, cinnamon and cloves. Set aside for a few minutes to allow chia to gel, then mix again with the whisk to break down any clumps.

5. Place in the fridge to allow to thicken for an hour before serving.

6. Store in the fridge in an air-tight, glass container for up to two weeks.

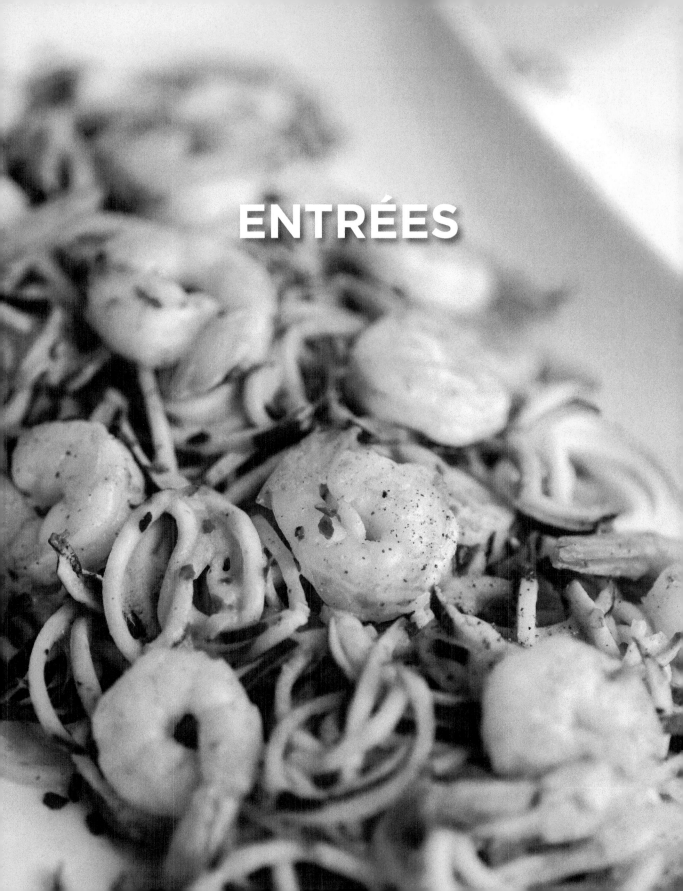

ENTRÉES

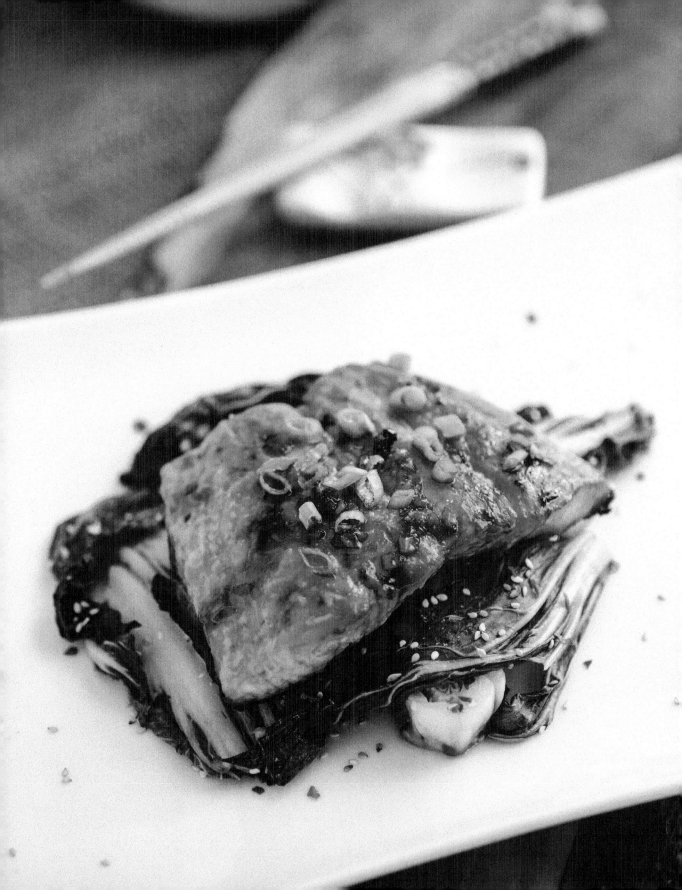

Super-Simple Asian Salmon

Serves 8

This dish has been a staple in my household since I was a child, and it's so flavourful and easy to make that it's on our menu at least once a week. Wild-caught salmon is high in omega-3 fats, which fight inflammation and do wonders for your brain health, making you both smarter and happier.

INGREDIENTS:

- 1 pound raw salmon, ideally wild
- 2 tablespoons liquid aminos
- 1 tablespoon avocado oil
- $^1/_2$ teaspoon sea salt
- $^1/_4$ teaspoon freshly-ground black pepper
- 1 tablespoon fresh dill

INSTRUCTIONS:

1. Preheat oven to 400°F.
2. Place the salmon on a baking pan.
3. Mix together liquid aminos and avocado oil, and pour over salmon. Sprinkle with sea salt, pepper, and fresh dill.
4. Bake for 15 to 20 minutes or until salmon flakes apart when pierced with a fork.

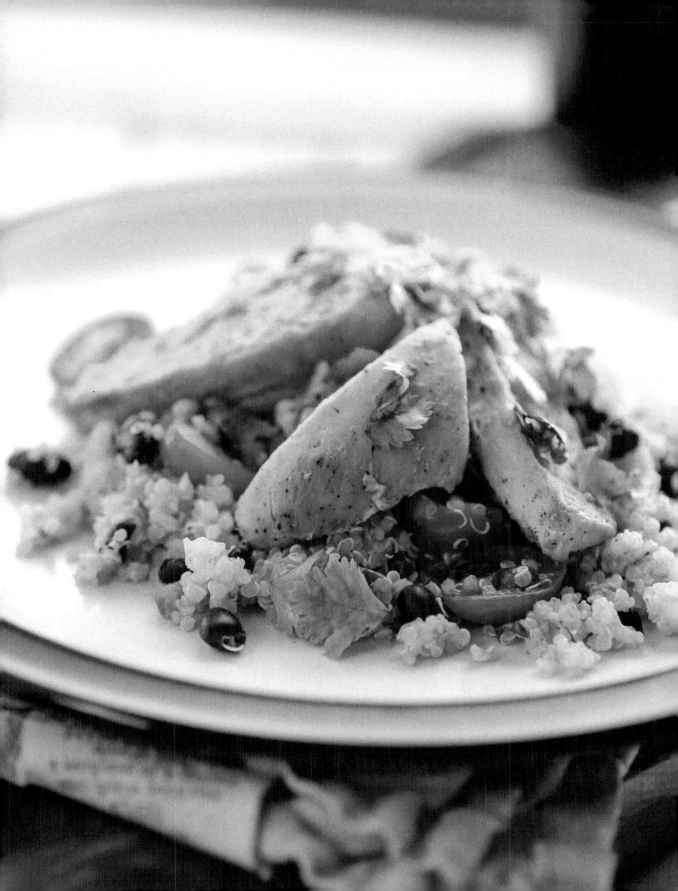

Cilantro-Lime Quinoa Bowl

Serves 4

This cilantro-lime quinoa bowl is simple to throw together and makes for an easy, satisfying, high-protein lunch or dinner. The cilantro and lime give this dish a zesty, delicious south-of-the-border flavour and provide the added detoxification benefits.

INGREDIENTS:

- 2 teaspoons extra-virgin olive oil
- 2 cups quinoa, rinsed thoroughly
- 4 cups vegetable broth
- 2 cloves garlic, minced
- 4 teaspoons ground cumin
- 1 teaspoon sea salt
- 1 (14-ounce) can black beans or chickpeas rinsed and drained
- $^1/_2$ cup freshly-squeezed lime juice
- 2 tablespoons extra-virgin olive oil
- a dash of cayenne
- 20 grape tomatoes, halved
- $^1/_2$ cup finely chopped red onion
- $^2/_3$ cup shredded romaine lettuce
- $^1/_2$ cup fresh cilantro
- 1 avocado, peeled and chopped
- optional: 2 cooked chicken breasts, cut into strips

INSTRUCTIONS:

1. Heat olive oil over medium heat in a medium-sized pan. Add quinoa and toast for about one minute or until no water remains on the quinoa. Add vegetable broth, garlic, cumin, and salt, and bring to a boil. Lower heat and simmer, covered, for 15 minutes.

2. Remove from heat, and let stand, covered, for five more minutes.

3. Remove lid, fluff with fork, then stir in black beans or chickpeas, lime juice, oil, cayenne, tomatoes, and onion.

4. Serve topped with lettuce, cilantro, avocado, and chicken breasts, if using.

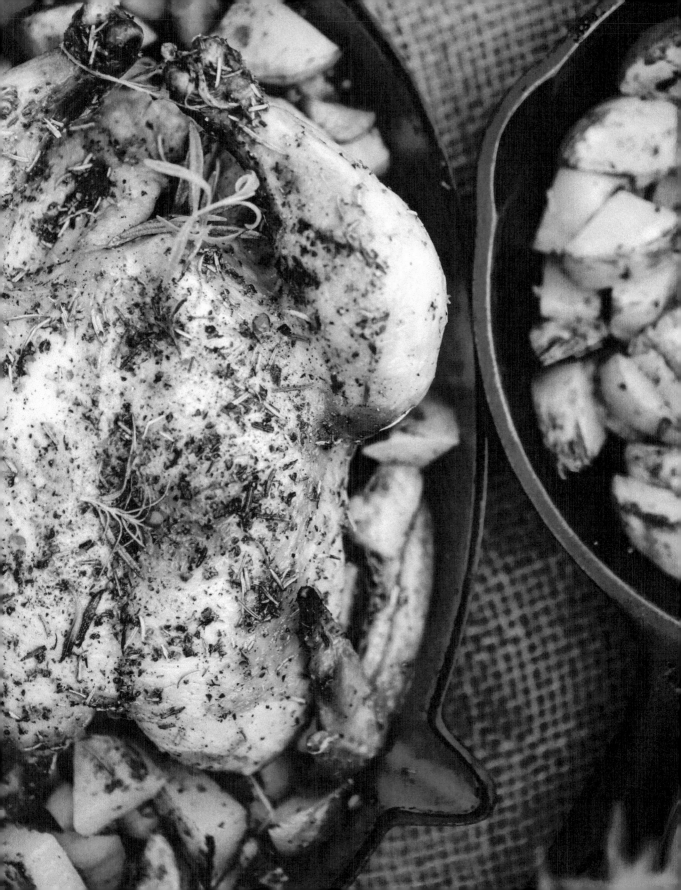

Perfect Herb-Roasted Chicken

Serves 4-6

This herb-roasted chicken recipe is on our menu at least once a week for the simple reason that it is SO DAMN GOOD! The different baking temperatures keep the skin crispy and the meat inside juicy. This dish is adored by both adults and children alike, and because it also helps build strong bones and muscles, it makes a great regular dinner staple.

INGREDIENTS:

- 1 whole organic chicken (weighing about 3 $^1/_2$ pounds)
- 1 tablespoon avocado oil
- 1 teaspoon dried basil
- 1 teaspoon dried thyme
- 1 teaspoon dried marjoram
- 1 teaspoon dried rosemary
- 1 teaspoon dried oregano
- 1 tablespoon sea salt
- $^1/_2$ teaspoon freshly-ground black pepper

INSTRUCTIONS:

1. Preheat oven to 425°F.
2. Rub avocado oil over the entire chicken.
3. Mix together all the herbs with the salt and pepper.
4. Rub the seasoning mixture into the chicken, then place the chicken in a roasting pan.
5. Cook the chicken in the pan, uncovered, for 20 minutes.
6. Lower the temperature and cook for another 60 minutes at 375°F, or until the juices run clear when pierced with a knife, or when the meat thermometer reaches 165°F.
7. Let stand for ten minutes before carving.
8. Reserve drippings and carcass for homemade chicken stock.

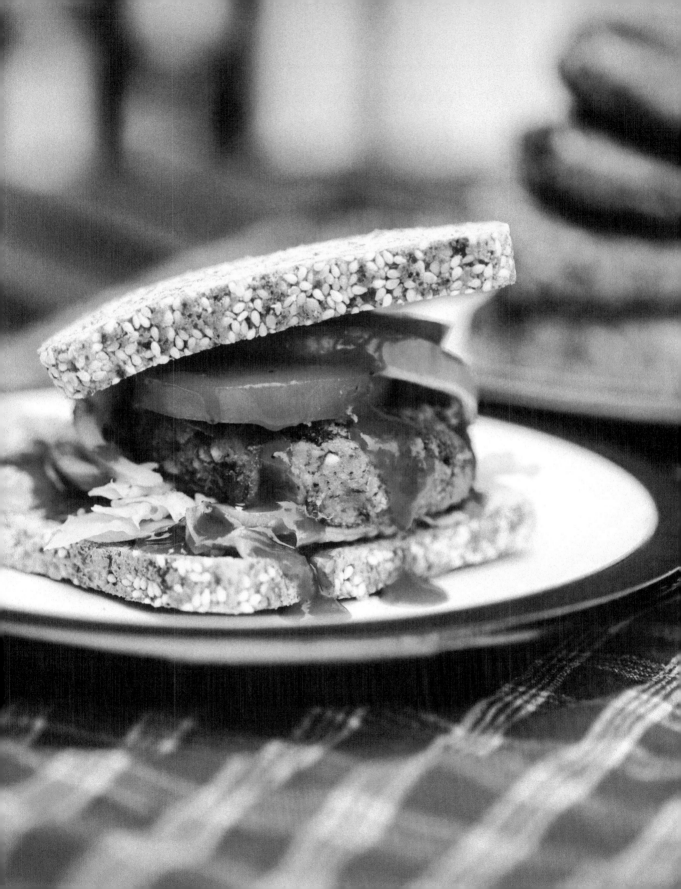

Nutty Bean Burgers

Serves 4–6

These healthy, hearty, and nutty meat-free burgers were the result of another one of my cooking mishaps. I had started making the Moroccan Yam Burgers from the Whitewater Cooks cookbook, and I got distracted and ended up leaving out a few key ingredients. When I tasted the batter, I realized how delicious it was. Now they are a part of our vegan rotation.

INGREDIENTS:

- 1 (14-ounce) can mixed beans, drained and rinsed
- 1 ¹/₂ cup mixed, unsalted nuts
- 2 garlic cloves, peeled and minced
- 1–2 teaspoons ground ginger
- 2 teaspoons ground cumin
- 2 tablespoons liquid aminos
- 2 tablespoons sesame oil
- 1 tablespoon ground flax
- 1 tablespoon chili powder
- 1 teaspoon ground coriander
- 1 teaspoon freshly-ground pepper
- ¹/₂ teaspoon ground cinnamon
- coconut oil, for cooking

INSTRUCTIONS:

1. Place all the ingredients, with the exception of the oil in a blender or food processor and pulse, so that the batter still has some texture.

2. Shape into patties the size of your palm. I suggest wetting your hands first, so that the batter doesn't stick to your fingers.

3. Cook the patties in a pan in coconut oil over medium heat for 5–10 minutes per side.

4. Serve atop a gluten-free bun or inside a romaine lettuce wrap along with your favourite toppings.

> **NOTE:**
> Inspired by Whitewater Cooks Moroccan Yam Burgers[45].

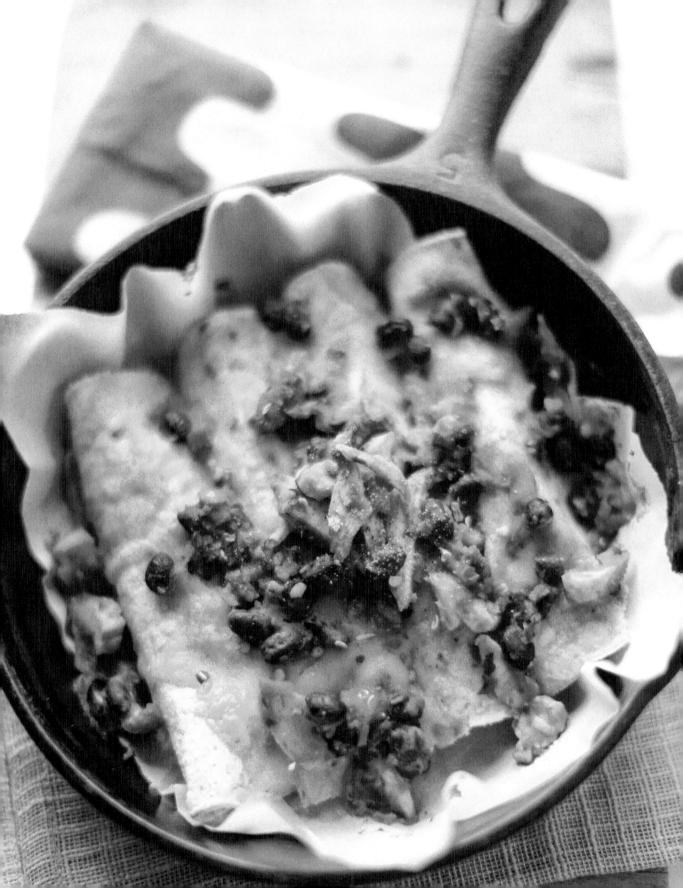

Spicy Chicken Enchiladas

Serves 4-6

Almost everyone I know loves enchiladas, but unfortunately, they are traditionally loaded with fat, calories, and excess sodium. Now, this family favourite is made over by replacing the cheese with butternut-squash purée and mashed black beans. For a quick weeknight dinner, prepare the butternut squash purée and chicken in advance.

INGREDIENTS:

- 1 tablespoon avocado or coconut oil
- $1/2$ cup white onion, peeled and chopped
- 1 teaspoon chili powder
- $1/2$ teaspoon ground cumin
- 1 cup butternut squash purée
- 1 cup salsa
- $1/4$ teaspoon sea salt
- 1 (14-ounce) can black beans, drained and rinsed
- 1 cup shredded chicken
- optional: 1 cup mozzarella-style dairy-free Daiya cheese
- optional: $1/4$ cup chopped fresh cilantro
- 6 gluten-free tortillas

INSTRUCTIONS:

1. In a medium saucepan, sauté onion in avocado oil until translucent. Add chili powder and cumin, and sauté for another minute or so.

2. Add butternut squash purée, salsa, and salt, and stir to combine. Add in the black beans and mash them down with a potato masher (it's okay if some whole beans remain).

3. Add the chicken and mix until well combined, then remove from heat.

4. Place about $1/2$ cup of chicken mixture in the middle of each tortilla, reserving about 1 cup of the mixture for later. If you are using the Daiya cheese and cilantro, sprinkle about $1/8$ cup cheese and 1 tablespoon of cilantro on each tortilla, then roll up them up, and arrange the tortillas seam-side-down in a ceramic baking dish.

5. Spoon reserved mixture over the top of the tortillas and, if using, sprinkle with leftover cheese. Broil on high heat for two to three minutes or until the cheese melts. Be careful that the wraps don't burn.

6. Serve immediately.

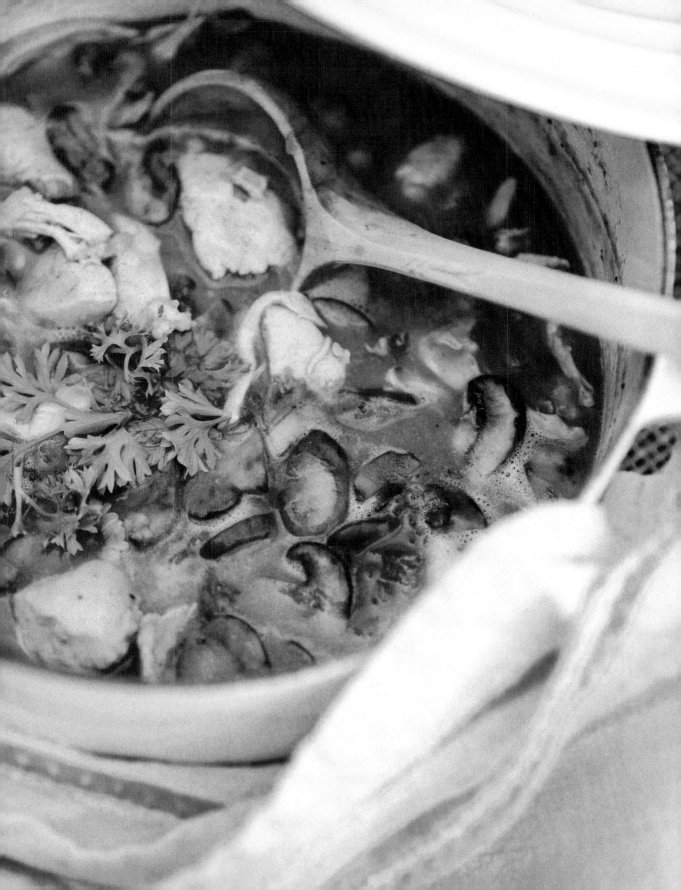

Super-Simple Pumpkin Chicken

Serves 4–6

This pumpkin-chicken recipe tastes incredibly creamy and flavourful, but even though it tastes decadent, the health powers of coconut and pumpkin make it a nutritional powerhouse of a meal. High in fibre, protein, and healthy fat, this meal will balance your blood sugar and keep you full for hours.

INGREDIENTS:

- 1 tablespoon avocado or coconut oil
- 4 uncooked chicken breasts, sliced into bite-sized pieces
- sea salt and freshly ground pepper, to taste (for chicken)
- 2 tablespoons coconut oil
- 2 cups sliced mushrooms
- 1 onion, peeled and chopped
- $1/2$ (796 ml) can pumpkin purée
- $1/2$ cup coconut cream, scooped off the top of a can of chilled, full-fat coconut milk
- $1/8$ teaspoon of ground nutmeg
- $1/2$ cup chicken broth
- 1 teaspoon arrowroot powder

INSTRUCTIONS:

1. Heat a frying pan over medium-high heat. Add oil to coat the pan, then add the chicken and cook until evenly browned (make sure no signs of pink are showing). Season with salt and pepper, then remove from heat, and set aside.

2. In a large pot, sauté mushrooms and onions in coconut oil for about five minutes or until the onions are translucent.

3. Add browned chicken, pumpkin purée, coconut cream, nutmeg, and chicken broth. While bringing to a boil, ladle a $1/4$ cup of the pumpkin-coconut sauce into a small bowl. Stir in the arrowroot powder until it dissolves, then add the mixture back into the pot.

4. Let simmer for about ten minutes, or until chicken is cooked through, watching the pot carefully so the coconut milk doesn't burn.

5. Serve over a bed of gluten-free noodles or rice.

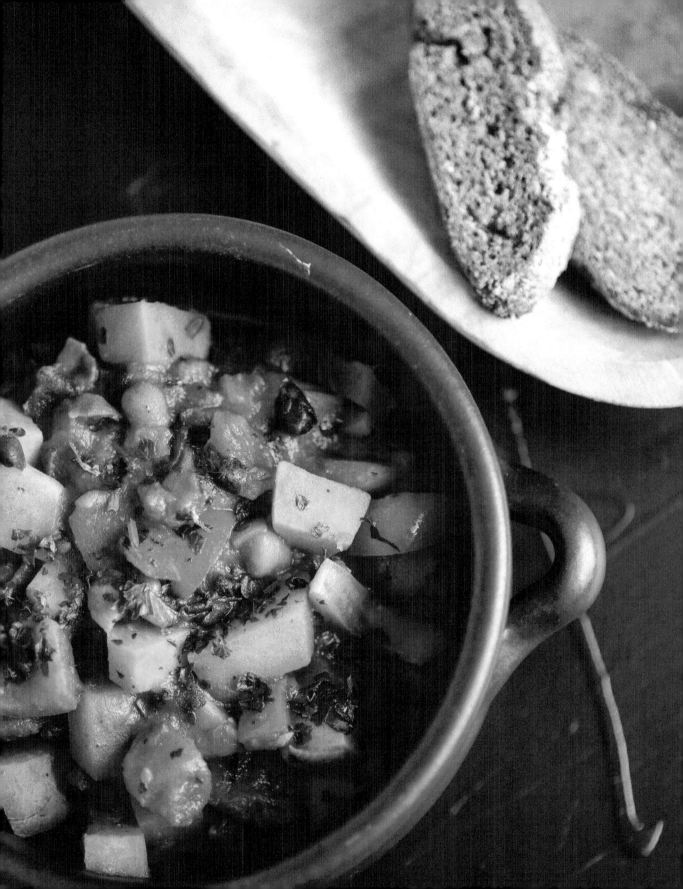

Vegan Sweet Potato Chili

Serves 6–8

You won't miss the meat in this nutritious Vegan Sweet Potato Chili and it's a great way to rack up your recommended daily servings of vegetables. Sweet potatoes and carrots pair perfectly with fall spices to create a depth of flavour that will have you reaching for seconds.

INGREDIENTS:

- 4 cups vegetable broth
- 1 cup organic pasta sauce
- 1 sweet potato, peeled and chopped
- 2 stalks celery, chopped
- 2 carrots, peeled and chopped
- 1 red bell pepper, chopped
- 1 (28-ounce) can crushed tomatoes
- 1 (14-ounce) can black beans, drained and rinsed
- 1 $^1/_2$ teaspoons ground cumin
- 1 teaspoon chili powder
- $^1/_2$ teaspoon ground coriander
- 1 $^1/_2$ teaspoons freshly-ground black pepper
- $^1/_2$ teaspoon dried oregano
- 1 teaspoon sea salt
- 1 tablespoon finely chopped, fresh parsley, for garnish

INSTRUCTIONS:

1. Pour vegetable broth into a large pot and bring to a boil.

2. Add remaining ingredients, reduce heat to low and simmer uncovered for 60 minutes, stirring occasionally to prevent the chili from burning.

3. Top with fresh parsley and serve immediately, or wait to eat it until the next day for an even greater depth of flavour.

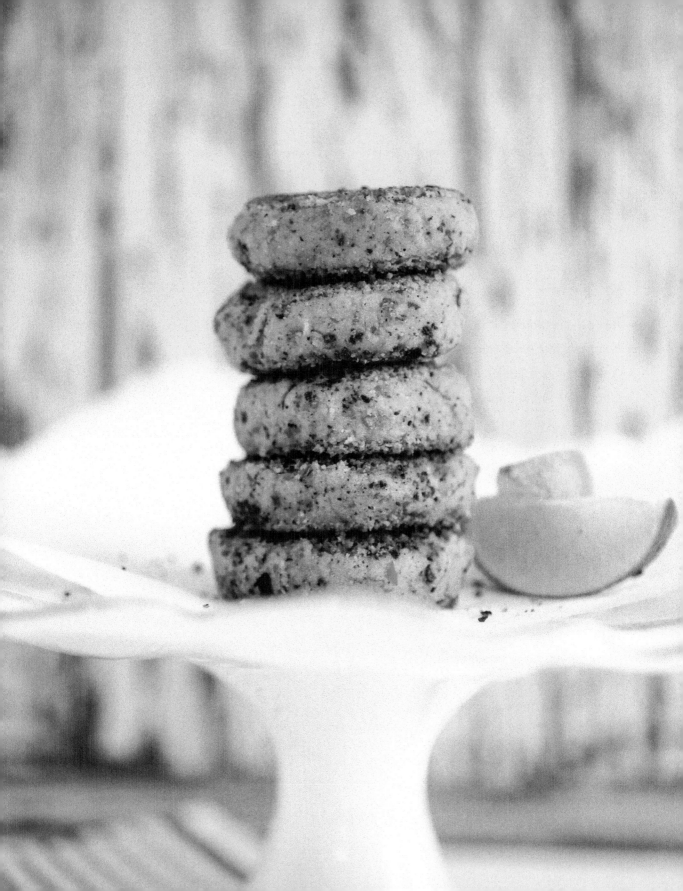

Vegan Falafel

Serves 4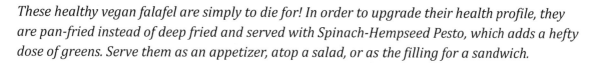

These healthy vegan falafel are simply to die for! In order to upgrade their health profile, they are pan-fried instead of deep fried and served with Spinach-Hempseed Pesto, which adds a hefty dose of greens. Serve them as an appetizer, atop a salad, or as the filling for a sandwich.

INGREDIENTS:

- 1 (14-ounce) can chickpeas, drained and rinsed
- $^1/_4$–$^1/_2$ red bell pepper, chopped
- 2 tablespoons gluten-free oat flour
- 2 tablespoons white rice flour
- 2 tablespoons buckwheat flour
- 1 teaspoon baking powder
- 2 tablespoons fresh cilantro leaves
- 1 tablespoon freshly-squeezed lemon juice
- $^1/_2$–1 teaspoon ground cumin
- 1 teaspoon garlic powder
- 1 teaspoon sea salt
- a pinch of cayenne
- avocado oil, for sautéing

INSTRUCTIONS:

1. Add all ingredients, with the exception of the avocado oil to a food processor and process until a dough forms. Form into two-inch wide patties.

2. Heat one tablespoon of oil in a frying pan over medium heat. Add as many patties as you can fit (allowing for space between each patty) and fry until golden brown on each side. Remove, and repeat with remaining patties.

3. Serve with the *Spinach-Hempseed Pesto* (from the *Sweet n Savoury Dips and Dressings* section) and enjoy immediately.

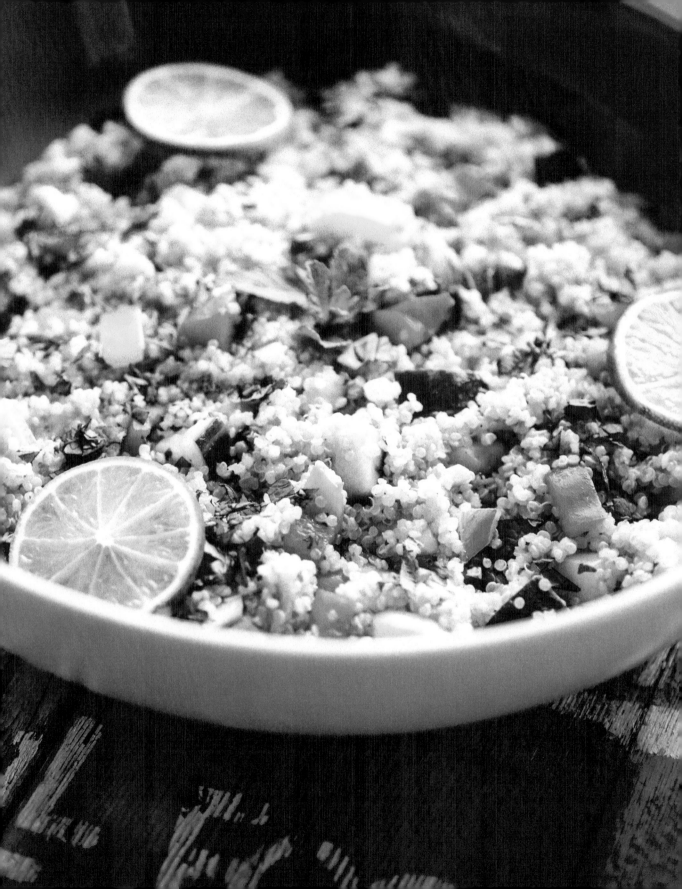

Fresh Quinoa Salad

Serves 8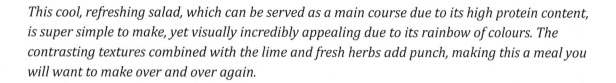

This cool, refreshing salad, which can be served as a main course due to its high protein content, is super simple to make, yet visually incredibly appealing due to its rainbow of colours. The contrasting textures combined with the lime and fresh herbs add punch, making this a meal you will want to make over and over again.

INGREDIENTS:

- 2 cups vegetable broth
- 1 cup quinoa, rinsed thoroughly
- $^1/_2$ red bell pepper, diced
- $^1/_2$ yellow bell pepper, diced
- $^1/_2$ medium red onion, peeled and diced
- $^1/_2$ English cucumber, peeled, seeded, and diced
- 2–3 tablespoons fresh mint, chopped finely
- juice of 1 lime
- 3–4 tablespoons extra-virgin olive oil
- sea salt and freshly-ground pepper, to taste

INSTRUCTIONS:

1. Pour the vegetable broth into a medium saucepan and bring to a boil.

2. Add the quinoa, cover, reduce heat to medium-low, and cook for approximately 15 minutes, or until all liquid is absorbed. Set aside to cool.

3. Add cooled quinoa to a large bowl along with the remaining ingredients, and mix until well-combined.

4. Top with a few lime slices and serve immediately.

> **NOTE:**
> This recipe was created by my good friend and dietitian, Ariadne Legendre, and is being printed with her permission.

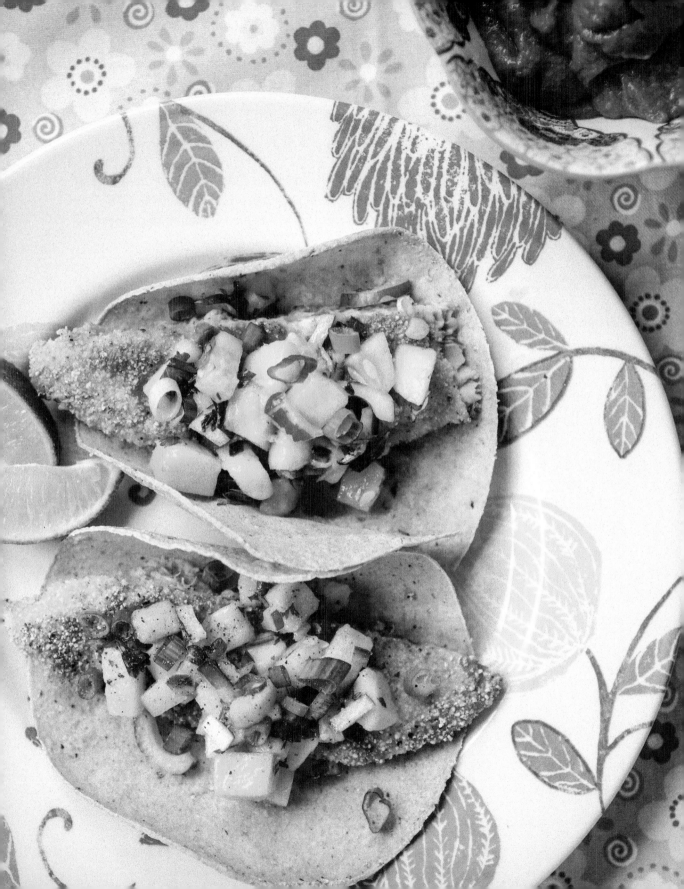

Fish Tacos

Makes 6 Tacos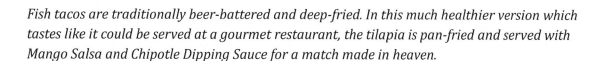

Fish tacos are traditionally beer-battered and deep-fried. In this much healthier version which tastes like it could be served at a gourmet restaurant, the tilapia is pan-fried and served with Mango Salsa and Chipotle Dipping Sauce for a match made in heaven.

INGREDIENTS:

- 1 large egg
- $1/3$ cup organic corn meal
- 2 x 6–8 ounce tilapia filets
- sea salt and freshly-ground pepper, to taste
- 2 tablespoons coconut oil
- 6 organic corn taco shells

INSTRUCTIONS:

1. Preheat oven to 400°F.
2. Crack the egg into a bowl and whisk until frothy, then pour onto a small plate.
3. Place the corn meal onto a separate plate.
4. Coat each tilapia filet in the egg and then the corn meal, and season both sides with salt and pepper.
5. Melt the coconut oil in a pan and fry each side of the filets for about two to three minutes on high heat and then another eight to ten minutes on low heat, until golden brown and cooked through.
6. Remove from heat, use a fork to separate into smaller pieces, and cover to keep warm.
7. Place corn taco shells on a baking sheet and bake for five minutes.
8. To assemble tacos, first add the tilapia to the taco, then the *Mango Salsa* and finally the *Chipotle Dipping Sauce* (both from the *Sweet n' Savoury Dips and Dressings* section), or alternatively, some organic hot sauce.
9. Garnish with fresh green onions and serve with wedges of lime.

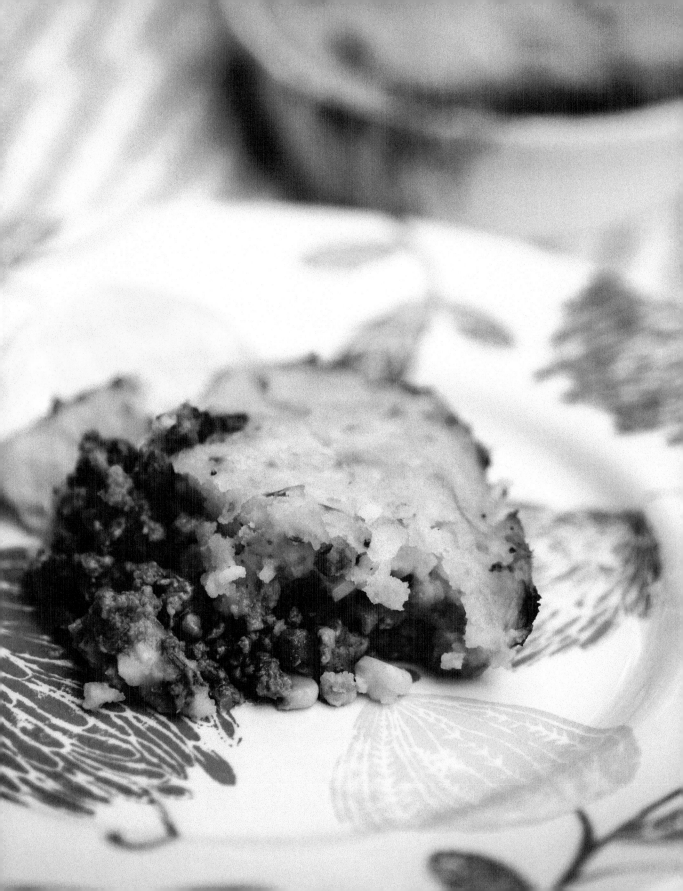

Healthy Shepherd's Pie

Serves 8–10

This updated Shepherd's Pie recipe eschews the heavy cream and butter in favour of a puréed Cream of Mushroom Soup (from the Soups, Salads and Sides section) making it lower in fat and much more nutrient-dense. Sub out the ground beef for ground turkey for an even leaner version of this recipe.

INGREDIENTS:

- 8 potatoes, peeled and chopped
- $1/4$ cup full-fat coconut milk
- 2 tablespoons coconut oil
- 2 teaspoons sea salt
- $1/4$ teaspoon freshly-ground pepper
- 2 $1/2$ pounds grass-fed ground beef (or ground turkey)
- $1/2$ tablespoon dried oregano
- $1/2$ tablespoon dried parsley
- $1/2$ tablespoon dried basil
- $1/2$ tablespoon sea salt
- $1/4$ teaspoon freshly-ground black pepper
- 2 cups homemade *Cream of Mushroom Soup* (from the *Soups, Salads and Sides* section)
- 1 cup frozen organic corn
- 1 cup frozen peas

INSTRUCTIONS:

1. Preheat oven to 370°F.

2. Bring potatoes to a boil in a large pot of water. Cook for 20 minutes or until you can easily pierce the potatoes with a fork.

3. Strain the water off the potatoes and mash potatoes along with coconut milk, coconut oil, sea salt, and pepper, until completely combined and smooth. Set aside.

4. Warm a large frying pan over medium-high heat. Add ground beef or turkey, breaking it apart into small pieces with a wooden spoon. Season with oregano, parsley, basil, sea salt, and freshly-ground black pepper. Continue to cook until evenly browned and no signs of pink are showing.

5. Drain meat and spread over the bottom of a deep baking pan. Pour mushroom soup over the beef.

6. Spread frozen corn and peas evenly over the top of the beef.

7. Top with mashed potatoes and bake for 30–35 minutes. Serve warm.

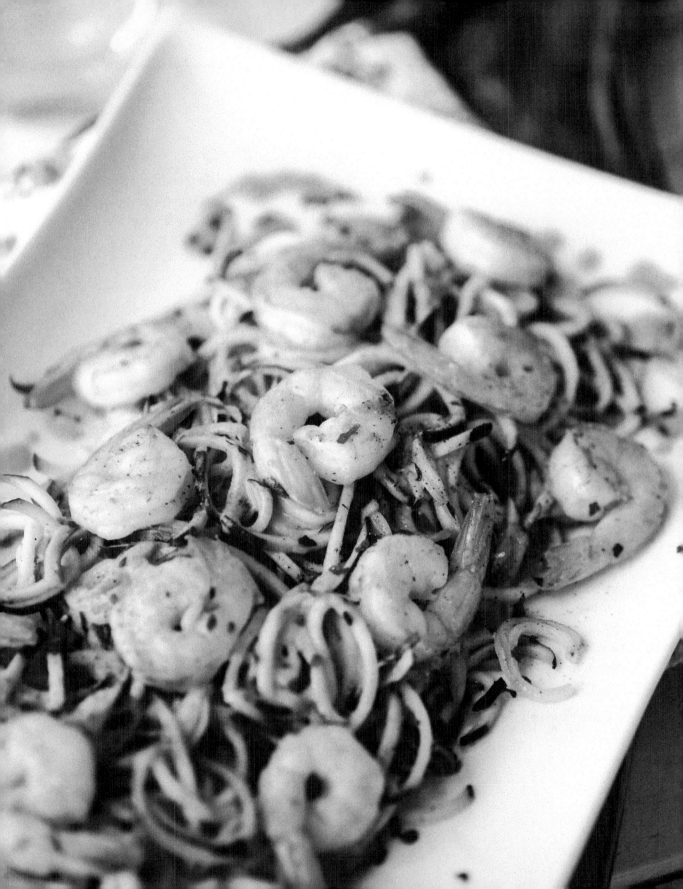

Zucchini Pasta with Shrimp in a Rosé Sauce

Serves 2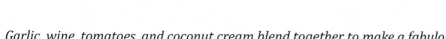

Garlic, wine, tomatoes, and coconut cream blend together to make a fabulous rosé sauce that will fill your home with the aromas of Italy. Substituting zucchini noodles for traditional white pasta decreases the carbohydrate load and provides added fibre and vitamin C.

INGREDIENTS:

- 2 tablespoons extra-virgin olive oil
- 12 jumbo-sized shrimp, uncooked, with tails on
- 1 garlic clove, peeled and minced
- ½ teaspoon sea salt
- ¼ teaspoon freshly-ground pepper
- ¼ cup dry white wine
- 2 tablespoons freshly-squeezed lemon juice
- 2 tablespoons coconut cream, scooped off the top of 1 can of chilled, full-fat coconut milk
- 1 tablespoon tomato paste
- ¼ teaspoon red pepper flakes
- sea salt and freshly-ground pepper, to taste
- 1 tablespoon extra-virgin olive oil
- 2 medium zucchinis, spiralized into zucchini noodles

INSTRUCTIONS:

1. In a large skillet, heat oil over medium-high heat. Add the shrimp, garlic, sea salt, and pepper. Cook, stirring frequently, until the shrimp turn pink and are cooked through, about three minutes. Using a slotted spoon, remove the shrimp and set aside.

2. Add the white wine, lemon juice, coconut cream, tomato paste, and red pepper flakes to the skillet. Bring the mixture to a boil. Reduce the heat to medium-low, and simmer for seven to eight minutes or until the sauce thickens.

3. Add the cooked shrimp to the skillet, season with salt and pepper, and set aside.

4. In a medium skillet, heat oil over medium-high heat. Add the spiralized zucchini and sauté for about 2–3 minutes. Place zucchini noodles into a serving dish, top with rosé sauce and shrimp, and serve.

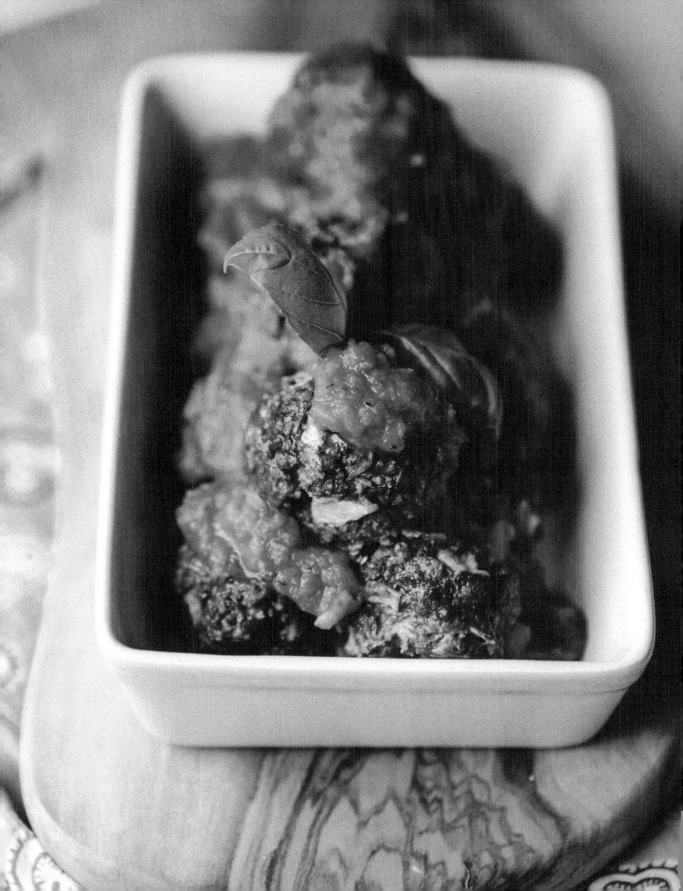

Sweet 'n' Sour Meatballs

Serves 6–8

You'll never want to buy store-bought meatballs again after you taste this dish! It's incredibly tasty, super easy to make, and your kids will adore the sweet flavour that the pineapple provides. Serve over rice or pasta as a complete meal or on its own as an appetizer.

INGREDIENTS:

Meatball ingredients:

- 1 teaspoon Chinese five-spice powder
- 2 teaspoons minced garlic
- ½ yellow onion, peeled and minced
- 2 pieces gluten-free bread, twice toasted and broken into pieces
- 1 teaspoon turmeric
- 1 teaspoon dried parsley
- 1 teaspoon sea salt
- 1 pound lean ground beef
- 2 large eggs

Sauce ingredients:

- 2 cups chopped, fresh pineapple
- $^1/_2$ cup marinara or pasta sauce
- 1 yellow onion, peeled and chopped
- 2 carrots, peeled and chopped
- $^1/_4$ cup organic ketchup
- 1 tablespoon raw honey
- 1 tablespoon apple cider vinegar
- 1 teaspoon sea salt

INSTRUCTIONS:

1. Preheat oven to 350°F.

2. To make meatballs, place the first seven meatball ingredients in a food processor and mix until a crumbly mixture forms.

3. In a large bowl, mix lean ground beef with the eggs and the bread-crumb mixture. Form into ping-pong sized meatballs.

4. Place meatballs on a pan and bake for 20–25 minutes or until no longer pink inside. Set aside.

5. To make the sauce, mix all sauce ingredients together in a food processor. Pour into a medium-sized pot and bring to a boil.

6. Once sauce starts to boil, reduce heat, and simmer for 15–20 minutes, covering with a lid.

7. Add the meatballs into the sauce and serve.

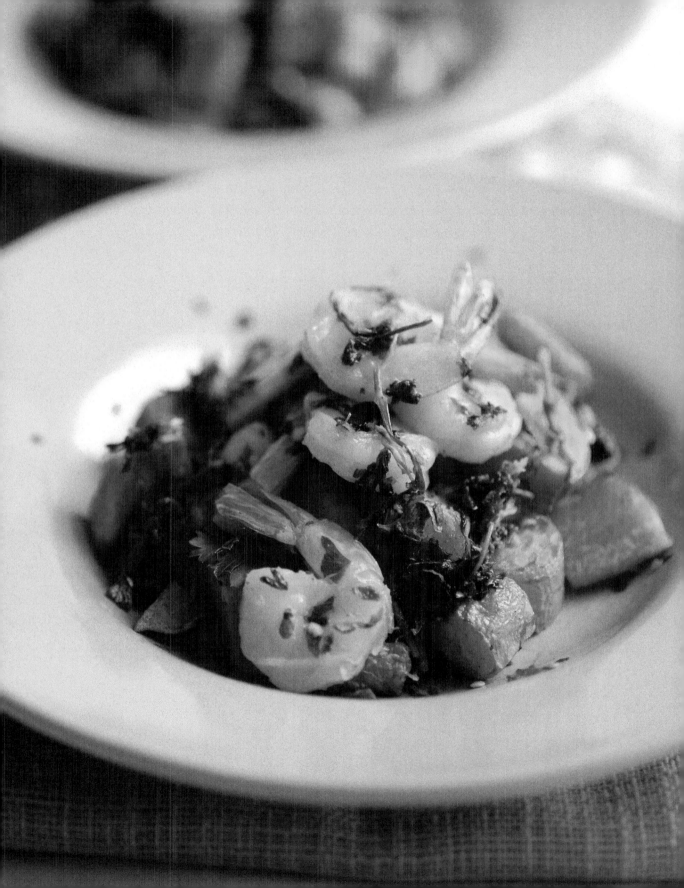

Shrimp with Parsley-Pesto Sauce

Serves 1–2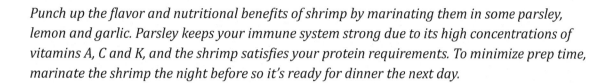

Punch up the flavor and nutritional benefits of shrimp by marinating them in some parsley, lemon and garlic. Parsley keeps your immune system strong due to its high concentrations of vitamins A, C and K, and the shrimp satisfies your protein requirements. To minimize prep time, marinate the shrimp the night before so it's ready for dinner the next day.

INGREDIENTS:

- 1 bunch Italian flat-leaf parsley, finely chopped
- juice of $1/2$ lemon
- 1 garlic clove, crushed
- 2 tablespoons extra-virgin olive oil
- $1/4$ teaspoon red pepper flakes
- $1/2$ teaspoon sea salt
- freshly-ground pepper, to taste
- 12 jumbo-sized shrimp, uncooked, with tails on
- 1 tablespoon avocado oil or grass-fed ghee

INSTRUCTIONS:

1. In a food processor, mix together the parsley, lemon juice, garlic, olive oil, red pepper flakes, sea salt, and pepper, until smooth.

2. Rinse shrimp well and pat dry with a paper towel.

3. Place shrimp into a medium-sized bowl, and pour the pesto over the shrimp, tossing until the shrimp is well-coated.

4. Place in the fridge to marinate for 30–60 minutes.

5. Add avocado oil to a skillet, set to medium-high heat. Add shrimp and cook about two minutes per side, or until the shrimp are cooked through and no longer translucent.

6. Serve alone as an appetizer, as a meal on top of pasta, or with the *Roasted Carrots and Sweet Potatoes* (from the *Soups, Salads and Sides* section).

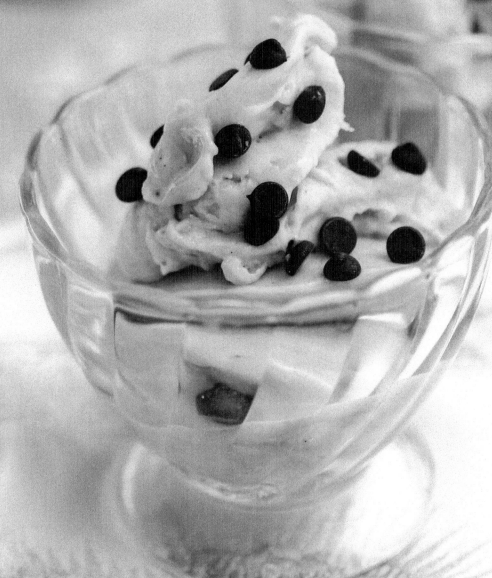

DESSERTS AND TREATS

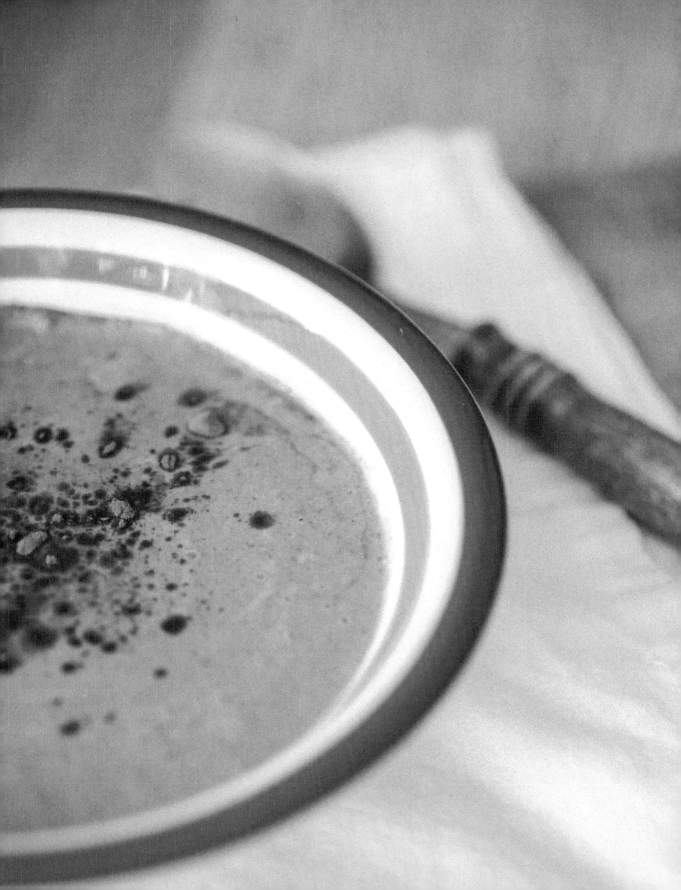

Chocolate Peanut Butter Pudding

Serves 1

A cross between a classic chocolate pudding cup and a Reese's peanut butter cup, this delicious pudding is sure to give you sweet dreams! Naturally high in complex carbs, tryptophan and magnesium, raw cacao and chia seeds are great for helping the body and mind relax, making this pudding a perfect night-time snack.

INGREDIENTS:

- $1/4$ cup warm water
- 1 tablespoon chia seeds
- 2 teaspoons raw cacao powder
- 1–1 $1/2$ tablespoons natural, unsweetened peanut butter
- $1/4$ cup and 2 tablespoons nut or seed milk
- $1/2$ banana, mashed
- $1/2$ tablespoon raw honey
- toppings: $1/2$ banana, chopped, and 1 tablespoon hemp hearts

INSTRUCTIONS:

1. In a medium-sized bowl, whisk together water with chia seeds and let sit for five minutes to thicken.

2. Whisk in remaining ingredients until well combined. Top with hemp hearts and sliced bananas.

3. Enjoy immediately (or if you like your pudding really thick, leave it in the fridge for a few hours), and enjoy chilled.

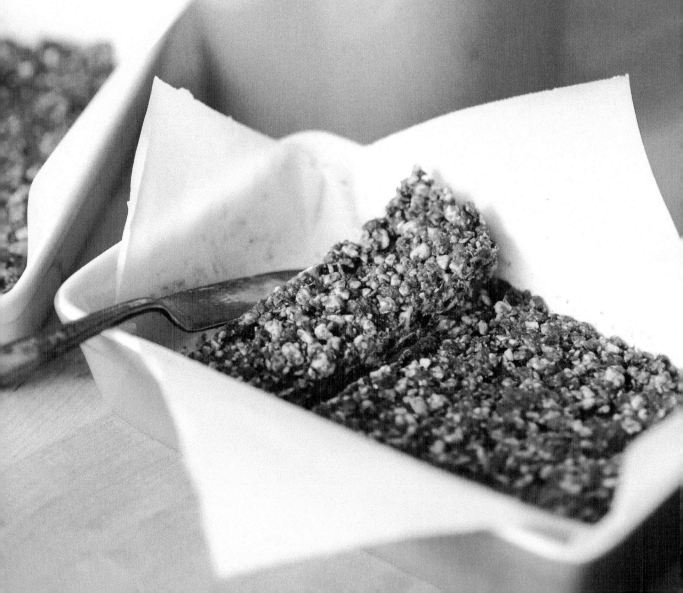

Perfect Granola Bars

Makes 30

These hearty, chewy, wholesome granola bars are the perfect portable snack. Full of healthy fats, fibre and protein, and yet sweet enough to taste like a real treat, they are sure to become a staple in your household.

INGREDIENTS:

- 1 cup slivered almonds
- $^1/_2$ cup sunflower seeds
- $^1/_2$ cup sesame seeds
- 6 cups quick-cooking, gluten-free oats
- 1 cup dried cranberries
- 1 cup raisins
- 1 cup raw honey
- 2 cups natural, unsweetened peanut butter
- 1 cup dairy-free chocolate chips
- $^1/_2$ cup coconut oil

INSTRUCTIONS:

1. In a food processor, mix almonds, sunflower seeds, and sesame seeds until semi-finely ground.
2. In a large bowl combine oats, cranberries, and raisins, then stir in the ground seed-and-nut mixture and set aside.
3. In a pot over low heat, melt together honey, peanut butter, chocolate chips, and coconut oil.
4. Remove mixture from heat and pour over the oat mixture. Stir until well combined.
5. Spread mixture onto a piece of parchment paper, flattening to desired thickness by placing another sheet of parchment paper on top and rolling with a rolling pin. Use a butter knife to make straighten out the edges and place into the fridge to cool for at least an hour.
6. Remove from fridge and cut into bars. Store in the fridge in an air-tight container for 3–5 days.

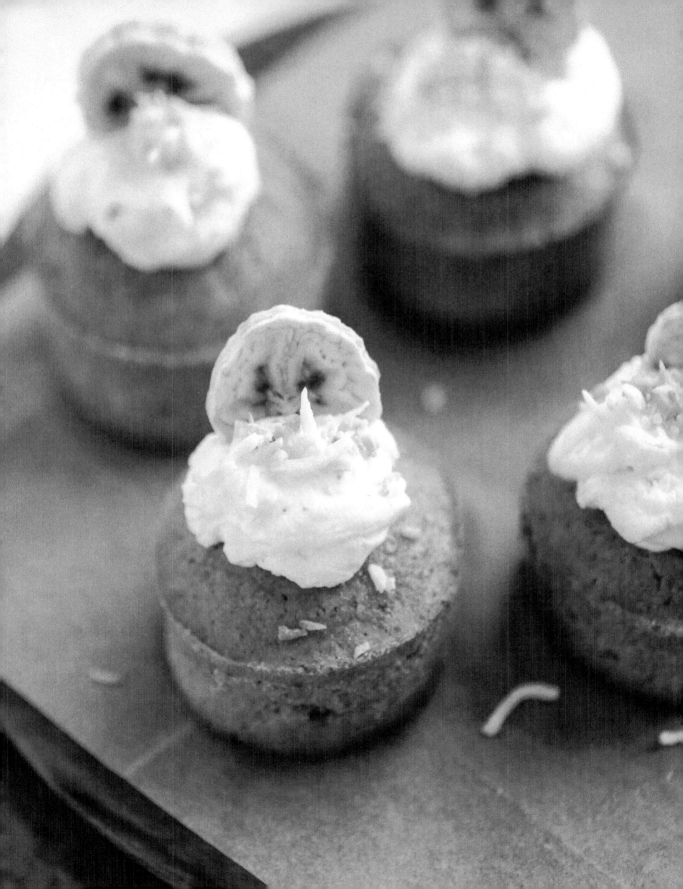

Hummingbird Muffins

Serves 12

Made with mood and energy-boosting whole grains, heart-healthy almonds, enzyme-rich pineapple, and electrolyte-dense bananas, these muffins will make your body hum in delight. Elevate these to cupcakes by topping with Coconut Whipped Cream or Cream Cheese Frosting.

INGREDIENTS:

- $2/3$ cup buckwheat flour
- $2/3$ cup gluten-free oat flour
- $2/3$ cup brown rice flour
- $1/4$ cup almond flour
- 1 teaspoon baking powder
- $3/4$ teaspoon sea salt
- $2/3$ cup raw honey
- $1/4$ cup fresh pineapple pieces
- $1/2$ cup ripe, mashed banana (about 1 large ripe banana)
- 2 large eggs
- 1 cup nut or seed milk (I used hemp)
- $1/4$ cup coconut oil, melted
- optional toppings: *Coconut Whipped Cream*

INSTRUCTIONS:

1. Preheat oven to 350°F.

2. Place flours, baking powder and sea salt into a food processor and mix together well.

3. Add in remaining ingredients and process until thoroughly combined.

4. Pour batter into muffin tins lined with silicone muffin liners, filling each about ¾ of the way full.

5. Bake for 30 minutes or until the muffins are firm to touch. If unsure, insert a toothpick into the middle of a muffin and remove. If the toothpick comes out clean, the muffins are ready.

6. Remove muffins from the muffin pan and let cool on a wire rack.

7. If desired, decorate each cupcake with a dollop of *Coconut Whipped Cream* (from the *Sweet n' Savoury Dips and Dressings* section) or *Cream Cheese Frosting* and top with a banana chip.

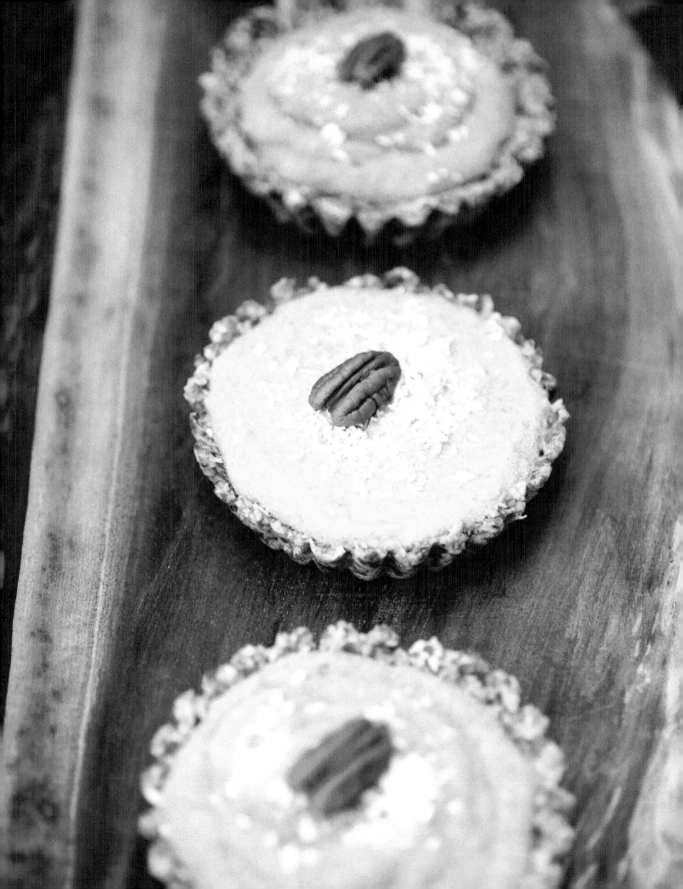

Raw Key Lime Pie

Serves 8

The cool, creamy, sweet and tangy key lime filling is contrasted with a nutty, caramel-like crust which will make you swoon. Although it tastes incredibly decadent, this pie is actually very healthy, and a far cry from the original version, which is traditionally made with condensed milk, butter, sugar and graham crackers.

INGREDIENTS:

Crust ingredients:

- $^3/_4$ cup pecans
- $^1/_2$ – $^3/_4$ cup shredded, unsweetened coconut
- a pinch of sea salt
- 8 Medjool dates, pitted

Filling ingredients:

- 4 avocados, peeled, pitted and quartered
- juice and zest of 2 large limes
- a pinch of sea salt
- 2 tablespoons raw honey
- 1 tablespoon tapioca starch
- $^1/_2$ cup coconut cream, scooped off the top of a can of chilled, full-fat coconut milk

INSTRUCTIONS:

1. To make the crust, blend all crust ingredients together in a food processor until the dough has a fine texture and sticks together when pinched between two fingers.

2. Press into the bottom of a round pie pan lined with parchment paper. Set aside.

3. To make the filling, blend together the avocados, lime juice, zest, sea salt, honey, and tapioca starch in a food processor. Set aside.

4. In your stand mixer, whip coconut cream until fluffy. Add the coconut cream into the food processor along with the avocado mixture and blend together.

5. Pour the filling into the prepared pie crust and freeze overnight, covered. Serve chilled.

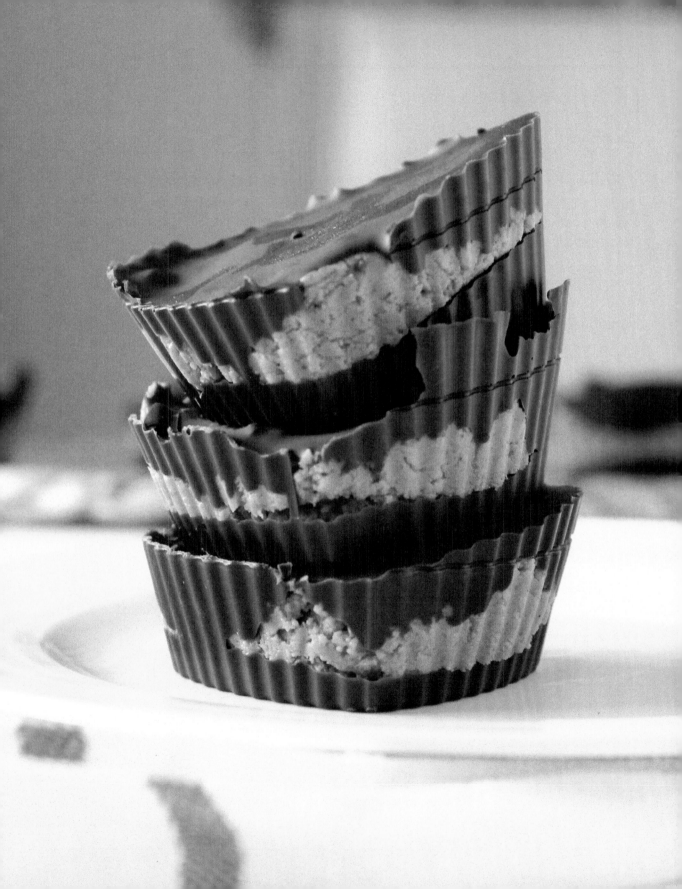

High-Protein Peanut Butter Cups

Makes 12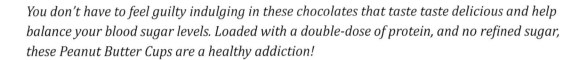

You don't have to feel guilty indulging in these chocolates that taste taste delicious and help balance your blood sugar levels. Loaded with a double-dose of protein, and no refined sugar, these Peanut Butter Cups are a healthy addiction!

INGREDIENTS:

- 1 10-ounce package dairy-free mini chocolate chips
- 1 tablespoon coconut oil
- a pinch of sea salt
- $^1/_2$ cup natural, unsweetened peanut butter
- $^1/_4$ cup raw honey
- 1 scoop (about $^1/_4$ cup) vanilla vegan protein powder

INSTRUCTIONS:

1. In a small pot, melt together the coconut oil and the chocolate chips over low heat, stirring regularly so the chocolate doesn't burn.

2. Once melted, stir in the sea salt, then remove from heat and pour about $^1/_2$ –1 tablespoon of chocolate into the bottom of each mini silicone muffin cup (or a 12-cavity silicone mold).

3. Place the silicone cups in the freezer to set for at least 10 minutes.

4. In the meantime, in a medium-sized bowl, mix together peanut butter, honey, and protein powder until smooth.

5. Remove the silicone cups from the freezer and place about $^1/_2$ tablespoon of the peanut butter filling in each mold. I usually roll the peanut butter filling into a ball and press it into the mold so it's nice and smooth.

6. Spoon another $^1/_2$ –1 tablespoon of melted chocolate on top and place into the freezer to set for at least an hour.

7. Pop the peanut butter cups out of the molds. To serve, let thaw for a few minutes before serving.

8. Store the rest in the freezer in an air-tight, glass container for up to two weeks.

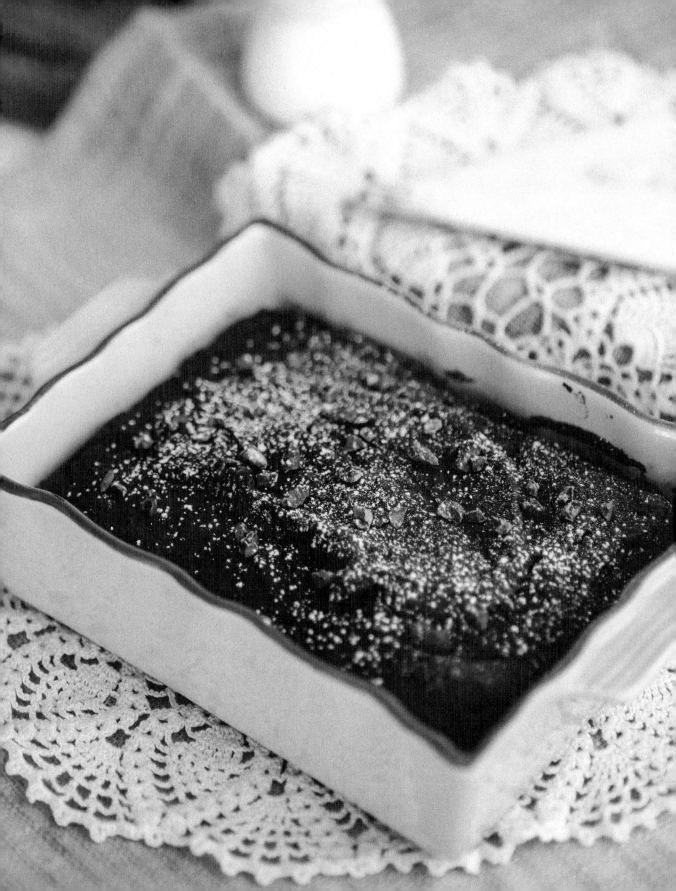

Triply Decadent Dark Chocolate Cake

Serves 10–12

Made with rich dark chocolate and creamy pumpkin, this cake will blow your mind, especially when served with the Coconut Whipped Cream. With significantly less fat and sugar than you would find in traditional cake, you won't feel guilty having one piece – or two.

INGREDIENTS:

- coconut oil, for greasing the cake pan
- $^1/_4$ cup hemp milk
- $^1/_2$ tablespoon apple cider vinegar
- 3 ounces 70% dark chocolate, finely chopped
- $^3/_4$ cup coconut oil, melted
- $^1/_2$ cup buckwheat flour
- $^1/_2$ cup brown rice flour
- $^1/_4$ cup almond flour
- 1 teaspoon baking powder
- 1 teaspoon baking soda
- $^1/_2$ teaspoon sea salt
- $^1/_2$ cup real maple syrup
- 1 $^1/_2$ cups pure pumpkin purée
- $^1/_2$ cup dairy-free dark chocolate chunks or chips
- optional: *Coconut Whipped Cream*

INSTRUCTIONS:

1. Preheat oven to 350°F. Grease a 9-inch round glass cake pan with coconut oil.

2. In a small bowl mix together hemp milk and apple cider vinegar and let sit for five minutes.

3. Meanwhile, in a small saucepan over low heat, melt together chocolate and $^1/_4$ cup of the coconut oil, stirring frequently so the chocolate doesn't burn. Set aside.

4. In a large bowl, whisk together flours, baking powder, baking soda and sea salt.

5. In a food processor, blend together the remaining $^1/_2$ cup coconut oil, maple syrup, hemp milk mixture, flour mixture, and pumpkin purée. Once well combined, pour in chocolate mixture and blend again until smooth. Mix in chocolate chunks by hand.

6. Pour batter into the greased cake pan and smooth out the top with a spatula. Bake for 40–45 minutes or until top is firm to a light touch.

7. Remove from oven and cool on a cooling rack before cutting. Serve warm with a big scoop of the *Coconut Whipped Cream* on top (from the *Sweet n' Savoury Dips and Dressings* section).

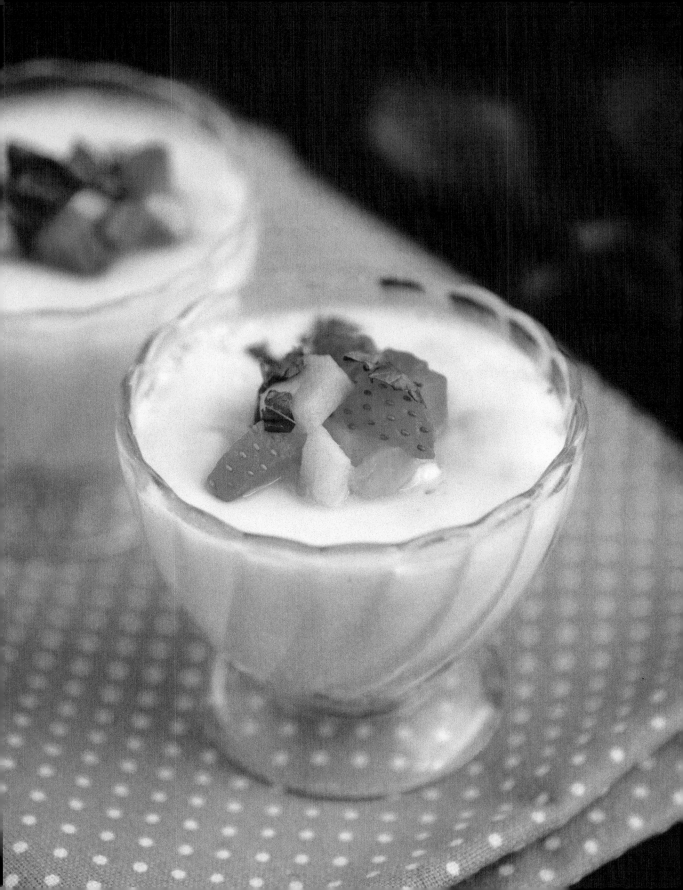

Coconut Panna Cotta

Serves 6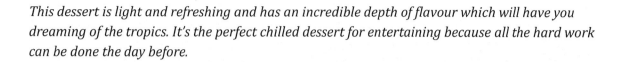

This dessert is light and refreshing and has an incredible depth of flavour which will have you dreaming of the tropics. It's the perfect chilled dessert for entertaining because all the hard work can be done the day before.

INGREDIENTS:

- 3 x 400 ml cans of full-fat coconut milk
- 2 envelopes of gelatin (about 2 $^1/_2$ teaspoons each)
- $^1/_2$ cup of raw honey
- seeds of 1 vanilla bean
- $^1/_2$ cup of finely chopped fresh strawberries
- $^1/_2$ cup of finely chopped mango (fresh or frozen will do)
- handful of fresh mint, finely chopped (or to taste)
- juice of 1 lime

INSTRUCTIONS:

1. In a small saucepan, mix together the coconut milk, gelatin, honey, and the seeds from the inside of the vanilla bean. Heat over medium heat until the gelatin is dissolved and milk is steaming.

2. Pour into small, individual bowls (to impress your guests, wine glasses work well, too).

3. Let cool in fridge for 4–5 hours.

4. In a small bowl, mix together strawberries, mango, mint, and lime juice and set aside.

5. When ready to serve, put one spoonful of the fruit mixture on top of each panna cotta.

NOTE:

This recipe was created by my good friend and dietitian, Ariadne Legendre, and is being printed with her permission.

TIP:

My favourite brand of gelatin is made by a company called Great Lakes. I like it because it's sourced from responsibly-farmed, pastured (grass-fed) animals as opposed to factory-farmed animals. You can find it here: http://greatlakesgelatin.com.

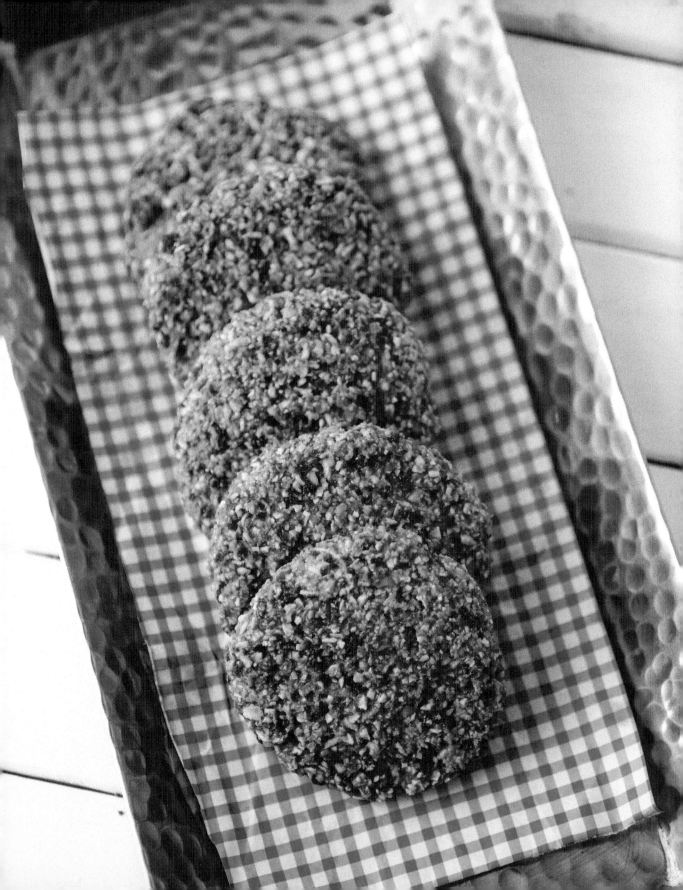

Oatmeal-Raisin Cookies

Serves 8–10

Incredibly low in sugar and made with minimal fat, these cookies make the perfect portable breakfast or snack to keep you energized for hours. Plus, they are super simple to make because all you have to do is throw all the ingredients together into a food processor and then bake them in the oven.

INGREDIENTS:

- 1 banana, peeled and chopped
- 1 cup gluten-free rolled oats
- $1/2$ cup walnuts
- 1 teaspoon pure vanilla extract
- $1/4$ cup brown rice flour
- $1/4$ cup sucanat or coconut palm sugar
- $1/4$ cup unsweetened applesauce
- $1/2$ cup shredded, unsweetened coconut
- a pinch of sea salt
- 1 teaspoon ground cinnamon
- $1/2$ cup raisins

INSTRUCTIONS:

1. Preheat oven to 350°F.
2. Add all ingredients to a food processor and blend until a dough forms.
3. Scoop out with a mini ice cream scoop (or use a tablespoon) onto a parchment-paper-lined cookie sheet. If desired, flatten slightly with the back of a fork.
4. Bake for ten minutes, then remove from the oven and cool on a wire rack.
5. Cookies can be stored in the fridge in an air-tight, glass container for 3–5 days.

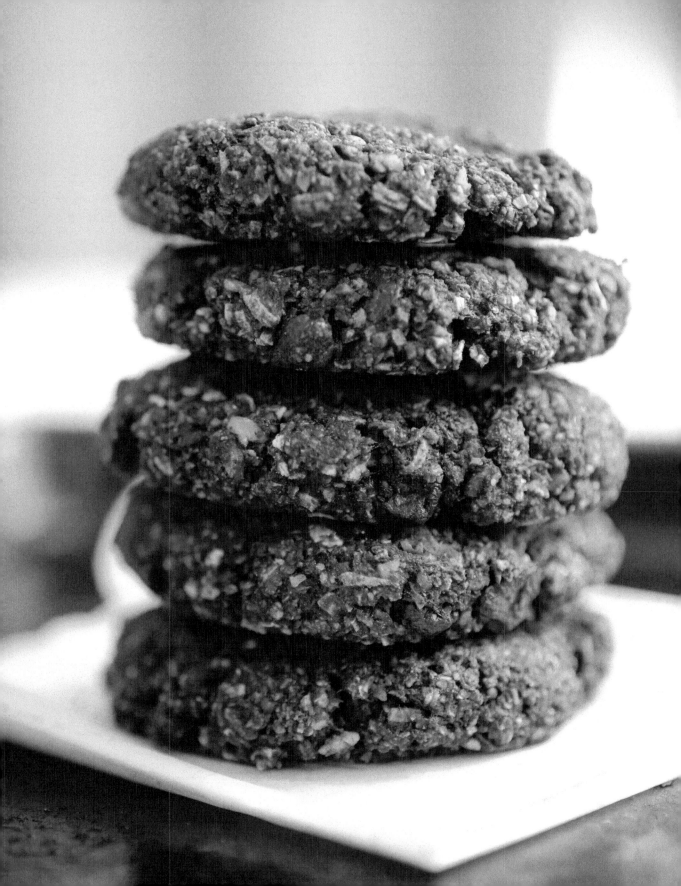

Cocoa-Banana Cookies

Serves 8-10

A perfect way to use up your over-ripe bananas, these vegan cocoa banana cookies have a lot of texture yet are incredibly moist. Made with wholesome, healthy ingredients, you can easily serve these for breakfast or a mid-afternoon snack.

INGREDIENTS:

- 2 ripe bananas, peeled and chopped
- 1 cup gluten-free rolled oats
- $^1/_2$ cup walnuts
- 1 teaspoon pure vanilla extract
- $^1/_4$ cup brown rice flour
- $^1/_4$ – $^1/_3$ cup sucanat or coconut palm sugar
- $^1/_4$ cup cocoa powder
- $^1/_2$ cup shredded, unsweetened coconut
- a pinch of sea salt
- 1 teaspoon ground cinnamon
- optional: $^1/_2$ cup dairy-free chocolate chips

INSTRUCTIONS:

1. Preheat oven to 350°F.
2. Add all ingredients, with the exception of the chocolate chips, to a food processor and blend until smooth.
3. Mix in chocolate chips by hand, if using.
4. Form into cookies (I like to scoop them out with a mini ice-cream scoop first) and place onto a parchment-paper-lined cookie sheet. If desired, flatten slightly with the back of a fork.
5. Bake for ten minutes, then remove from oven and let cool on a wire rack.
6. Store in the fridge in an air-tight, glass container for 3–5 days.

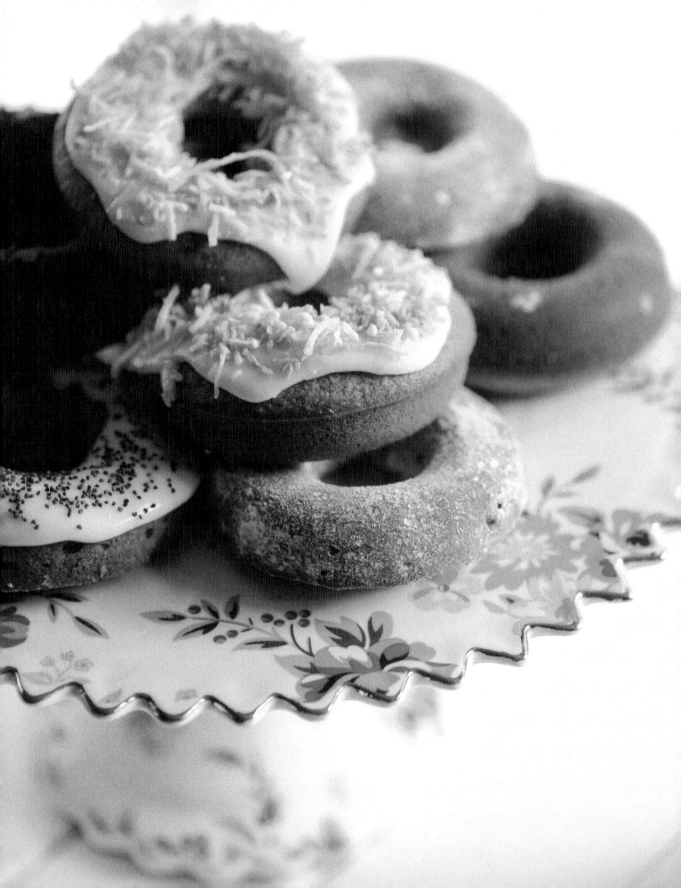

Banana Doughnuts

Serves 6

There is no problem letting the kids have doughnuts for breakfast when you can serve them this incredibly healthy alternative to the traditional, sugar-laden, deep-fried version. For added sweetness, top them with the sweet Coconut Lime Glaze and let them melt in your mouth.

INGREDIENTS:

Doughnut ingredients:

- $^1/_2$ cup gluten-free oat flour
- $^1/_2$ cup brown rice flour
- $^3/_4$ cup walnut pieces
- 2 teaspoons baking powder
- $^1/_2$ teaspoon sea salt
- 1 teaspoon ground cinnamon
- $^1/_2$ teaspoon ground nutmeg
- $^1/_3$ cup melted coconut oil
- $^1/_2$ cup coconut palm sugar
- 1 large egg
- 1 teaspoon pure vanilla extract
- $^1/_3$ cup mashed banana
- $^1/_2$ cup unsweetened almond milk

Glaze ingredients (optional):

- 1 cup gluten-free, organic icing sugar
- 1 tablespoon full-fat coconut milk
- 1–1 $^1/_2$ teaspoons freshly-squeezed lime juice

Topping ingredients (optional):

- ¼ cup toasted, shredded, unsweetened coconut

INSTRUCTIONS:

1. To make doughnuts, preheat oven to 350°F.

2. In a food processor, mix together flours, nuts, baking soda, salt, cinnamon, and nutmeg.

3. Add in coconut oil, sugar, egg, vanilla, mashed banana, and almond milk, and mix until thoroughly combined.

4. Pour into a doughnut pan and bake for 10-12 minutes, or until firm to the touch.

5. Cool on a wire rack and serve as it or top with the *Coconut Lime Glaze.*

6. To make glaze, mix together icing sugar, coconut milk, and lime juice in a stand mixer.

7. Pour half of the glaze into a small bowl, and save the rest for a second batch of doughnuts.

8. Dip each doughnut into the glaze and then sprinkle with the toasted coconut.

9. Store in the fridge in an air-tight, glass container for 3–5 days.

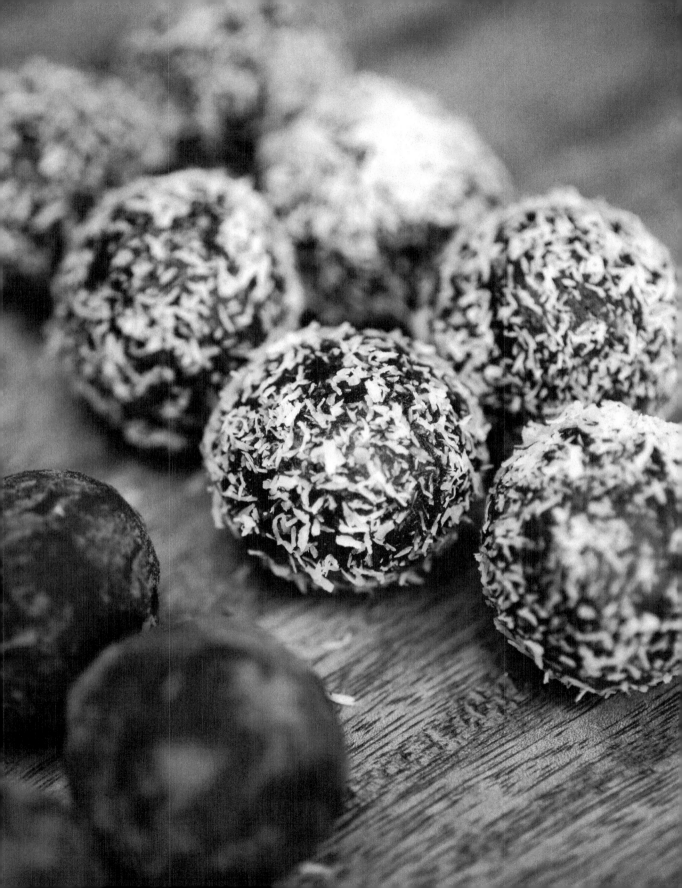

Raw Superfood Energy Balls

Makes 12 large balls

You would never know that these raw superfood energy balls contain a hefty serving of greens. Take these potent little balls of energy along with you on your active adventures, or pop a few in your mouth during a mid-afternoon slump, or whenever your immune system needs an extra boost.

INGREDIENTS:

- 1 scoop gluten-free greens powder
- ½ cup almond butter
- 4 Medjool dates
- ¼ cup real maple syrup
- ½ cup raw cacao powder
- ¼ cup hemp hearts
- ¼ cup sesame seeds
- 1 cup walnuts
- 1 teaspoon pure vanilla extract

INSTRUCTIONS:

1. Add all ingredients to a food processor and blend until a dough forms.

2. Roll into bite-sized balls. If desired, roll in shredded coconut, hemp hearts, or raw cacao powder.

3. Eat immediately or store in fridge in an air-tight, glass container for 3–5 days.

> **NOTE:**
> My favourite greens powder is Greens+ O which is made by *Genuine Health*. It is gluten-free and the purest, and most research-backed greens powder on the market. I also love that they have a fermented version!

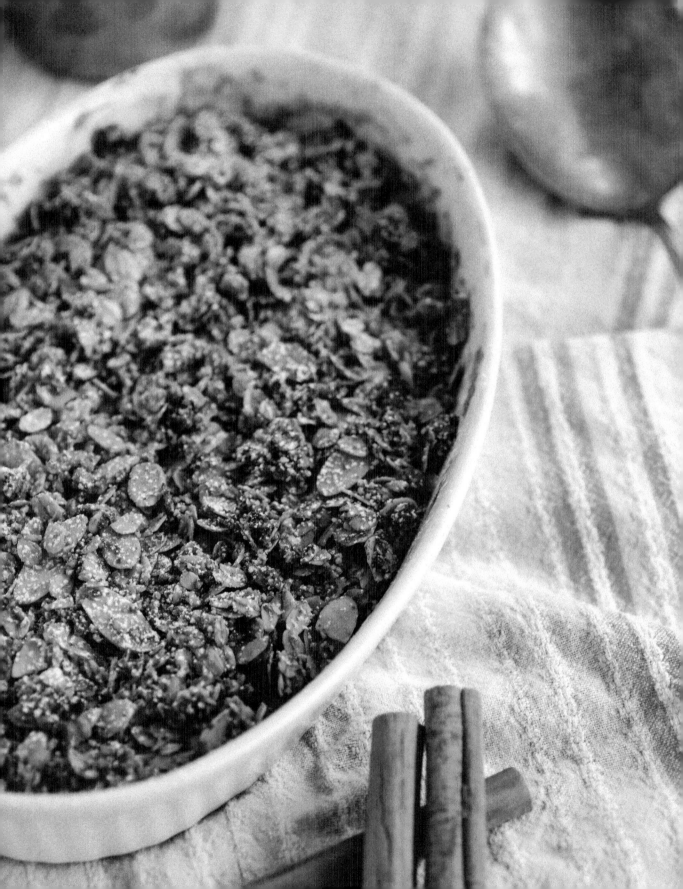

Apple Crisp

Serves 6-8

Warm sweet apples topped with a crispy, crumbly, oat and almond topping make this dessert as wholesome as it is delicious. The smell of baked apples and oats, along with cinnamon and nutmeg, will have everyone running to the kitchen.

INGREDIENTS:

Apple filling ingredients:

- 6 granny smith apples, peeled and sliced
- 2 tablespoons freshly-squeezed lemon juice
- 2 tablespoons fresh apple cider (or freshly-squeezed orange juice)
- $1/4$ cup coconut palm sugar
- 1 tablespoon arrowroot powder
- 1 teaspoon ground cinnamon
- $1/2$ teaspoon ground nutmeg

Crumble ingredients:

- 5 tablespoons coconut oil, melted
- 1 cup gluten-free, rolled oats
- $1/2$ cup sliced almonds
- $3/4$ cup almond flour or meal
- 2 tablespoons coconut palm sugar
- 2 tablespoons real maple syrup
- $1/2$ teaspoon sea salt
- 1 teaspoon ground cinnamon

INSTRUCTIONS:

1. To make filling, preheat oven to 375°F.
2. Place the apples in large bowl.
3. Mix together all other filling ingredients in a separate bowl, then pour over the apples.
4. Spread apples evenly over the bottom of a square 8 x 8 inch pan and bake for ten minutes.
5. In the meantime, mix together all topping ingredients with your hands untill thoroughly combined.
6. Remove apples from oven and turn up the heat to 400°F.
7. Sprinkle crumble mixture evenly over the apples and bake for 20 more minutes.
8. Remove from oven, and serve warm with a dollop of *Coconut Whipped Cream* (from the *Sweet n' Savoury Dips and Dressings* section).

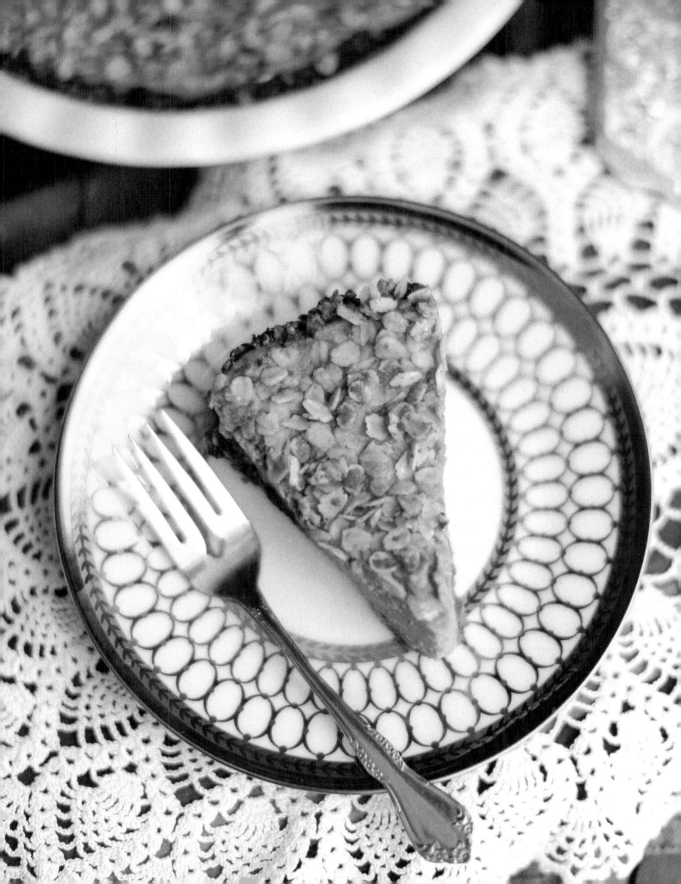

Sweet Potato Pie

Serves 8–10

Sweet-potato pie is a great alternative to traditional pumpkin pie. Slightly sweeter and earthier, and full of vitamins, antioxidants, and fibre, this pie is truly addictive. Bring it to your next party, and you are sure to be everyone's favourite guest!

INGREDIENTS:

Topping ingredients:

- 2 tablespoons coconut palm sugar
- 2 tablespoons coconut oil
- $^1/_2$ cup gluten-free rolled oats

Crust ingredients:

- 1 $^1/_4$ cups hazelnuts
- $^1/_2$ cup almond meal
- 1 $^1/_4$ cups pitted dates
- 1 teaspoon ground cinnamon
- a pinch of sea salt

Filling ingredients:

- 2 $^3/_4$ cups cooked, mashed sweet potato
- $^1/_2$ cup coconut cream, scooped off the top of 1 can of chilled, full-fat coconut milk
- 3 large eggs
- $^1/_4$ cup coconut oil, melted
- $^1/_2$ cup real maple syrup
- $^1/_4$ teaspoon ground nutmeg
- $^1/_4$ teaspoon ground cloves
- 2 teaspoons ground cinnamon

INSTRUCTIONS:

1. Preheat oven to 350°F.
2. In a small bowl, mix together all the topping ingredients, and then set aside.
3. In a food processor, mix together all the crust ingredients until they start to stick together.
4. Press the crust into the bottom and up the sides of a round, glass pie dish and set aside.
5. Mix all filling ingredients together in a food processor.
6. Pour the filling over the pie crust, then sprinkle with the topping.
7. Bake for 45 minutes, or until the filling is set.
8. Let cool, then place in fridge to set for at least an hour.
9. Serve with *Coconut Whipped Cream* (from the *Sweet n' Savoury Dips and Dressings* section).

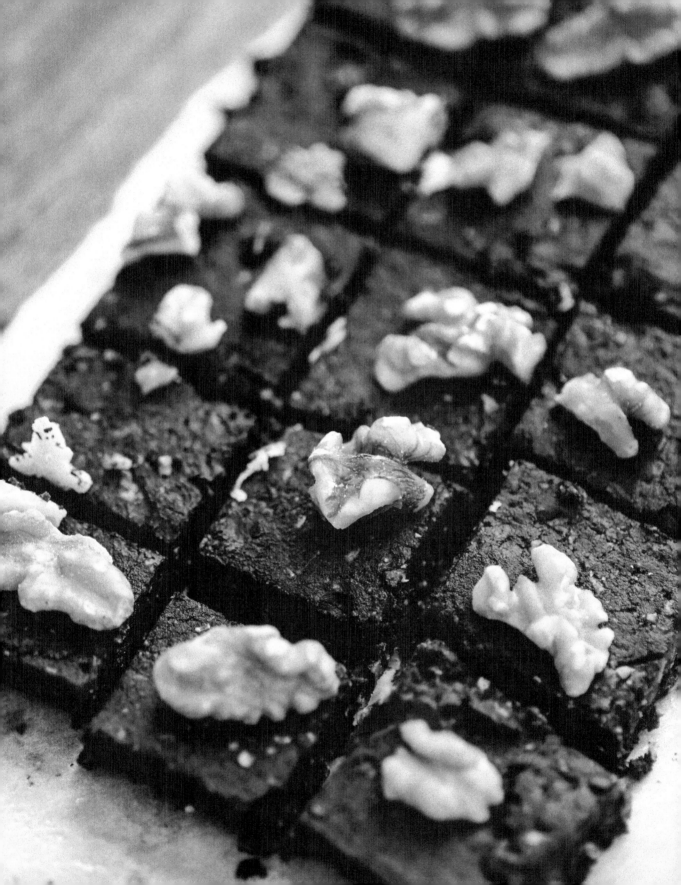

Raw Chocolate Brownies

Serves 12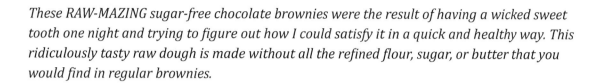

These RAW-MAZING sugar-free chocolate brownies were the result of having a wicked sweet tooth one night and trying to figure out how I could satisfy it in a quick and healthy way. This ridiculously tasty raw dough is made without all the refined flour, sugar, or butter that you would find in regular brownies.

INGREDIENTS:

- $^1/_2$ cup raw cacao powder
- 1 $^1/_2$ cups pitted Medjool dates
- $^1/_2$ cup cashew butter
- $^1/_4$ cup almond butter
- $^1/_2$ cup unsweetened coconut flakes
- $^1/_4$ cup unsweetened vanilla almond milk

INSTRUCTIONS:

1. Add all ingredients to a food processor and mix until a dough forms and no large chunks remain.

2. Press the dough down firmly into an 8 x 8 inch parchment-paper-lined pan. Smooth the top with a spatula or rolling pin.

3. Place in the fridge and let chill for about an hour before removing and cutting into 12 small squares.

4. Store in the fridge in an air-tight, glass container for 3–5 days.

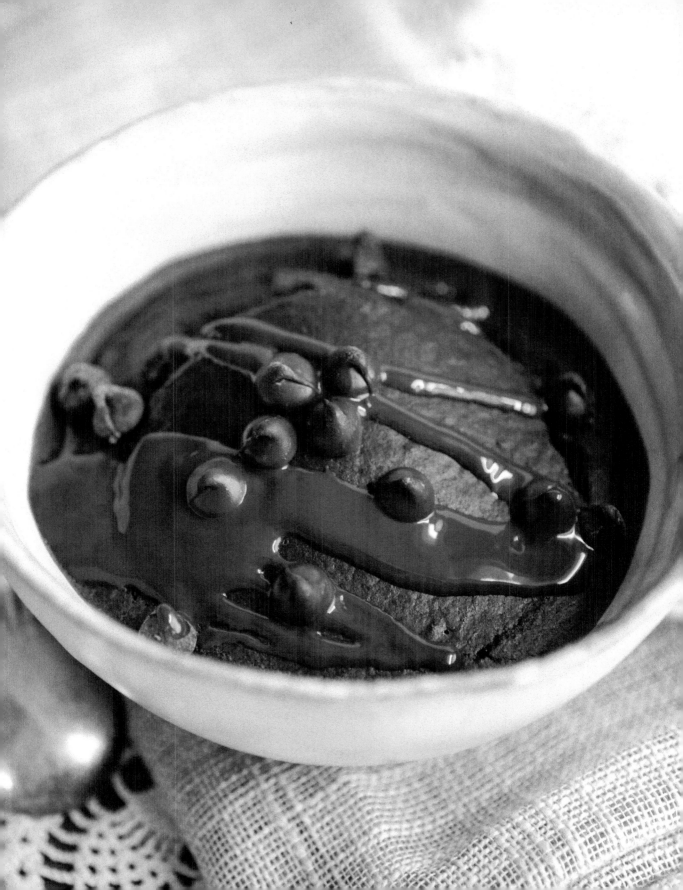

Chocolate Mug Cake

Serves 1–2

This cake is the result of needing a gluten-free, dairy-free alternative to send to school with my daughter for a classroom birthday celebration. It is quick and easy to make, and because it only serves one, you don't need to worry about being tempted by leftovers.

INGREDIENTS:

Icing ingredients:
- $1/2$ cup dairy-free mini chocolate chips
- 1 tablespoon coconut oil

Cake ingredients:
- 3 tablespoons gluten-free flour
- 2 tablespoons cocoa powder
- 2 tablespoons coconut palm sugar
- $1/4$ teaspoon ground cinnamon
- $1/4$ teaspoon baking powder
- 1 tablespoon unsweetened apple sauce
- 3 tablespoons unsweetened vanilla almond milk
- 1 large egg

INSTRUCTIONS:

1. To make the icing, melt together the chocolate chips and coconut oil in a double boiler (or carefully in a pot on the stove over low heat, making sure to stir the entire time so it doesn't burn).

2. Once melted, stir well, and set aside to cool while the cake bakes.

3. To make the cake, preheat oven to 350°F.

4. Mix all dry ingredients together thoroughly in an oven-safe mug.

5. Add in remaining ingredients and mix again, making sure no dry spots remain.

6. Place mug in the oven and bake for 25–27 minutes, or until cooked through.

7. Remove the mug from the oven with a dishcloth or glove mitt, and then tip the mug over and empty cake onto a wire baking rack to cool.

8. Frost cake with icing and serve.

> **NOTE:**
> Although I don't recommend microwaving regularly, if you are in a time crunch, this mug cake can be cooked in the microwave for 2-3 minutes instead of being baked for 25 minutes.

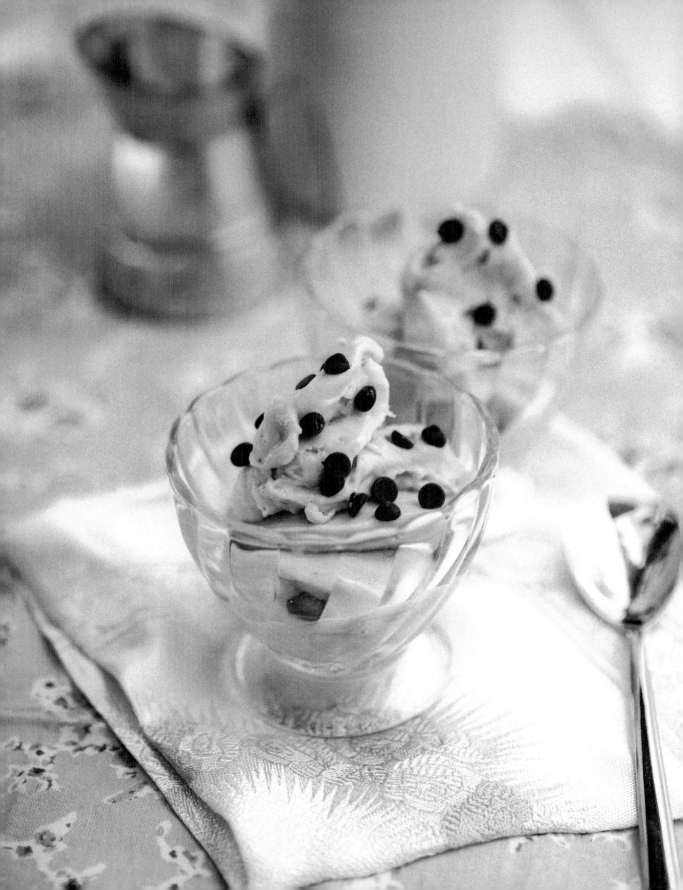

Chocolate-Peanut-Butter Ice Cream

Serves 2

When mixed with the right ingredients, frozen bananas can easily satisfy your cravings for ice cream without any of the guilt. I usually keep a huge batch of bananas in the freezer so that I can quickly whip up some 'nice cream' whenever the mood strikes.

INGREDIENTS:

- 2 frozen, ripe bananas, peeled and chopped
- 2 tablespoons natural peanut or almond butter
- 2 tablespoons coconut milk, from a carton
- 2 tablespoons raw cacao powder
- 1 teaspoon pure vanilla extract
- 1 teaspoon real maple syrup

INSTRUCTIONS:

1. Place all ingredients in your food processor and blend until smooth. You may need to scrape down the sides of the bowl several times.

2. Scoop into bowls, add your favorite toppings, (like the *Raw Vegan Caramel Sauce* from the *Sweet n' Savoury Dips and Dressings* section) and enjoy immediately.

Peanut-Butter Energy Balls

Makes 12

These three-ingredient peanut butter energy balls could not be any simpler! Packed with protein, fibre, heart-healthy fats, antioxidants and B vitamins, these treats are great for active families who are always on the go.

INGREDIENTS:

- 1 cup unsalted, unroasted peanuts
- 15 Medjool dates, pitted
- $1/4$ teaspoon sea salt

INSTRUCTIONS:

1. Add all ingredients to a food processor and mix until a dough starts to form.
2. Roll into ping-pong sized balls.
3. Store in the fridge in an air-tight, glass container for 3–5 days.

TIP:
Peanuts have the highest protein content of any nut, with 7.3 grams per ounce, which makes them an excellent plant-based protein source.

Lemon-Drop Energy Balls

Makes 12-14

These potent little lemony cancer-fighters are my favourite treat in this book. They taste just divine and are naturally high in minerals, antioxidants, vitamin C, fibre, and heart-healthy fats, making them the perfect snack for any time of day! Pop one, or two, or three!

INGREDIENTS:

- 1 $^1/_4$ – 1 $^1/_2$ cups raw cashews
- 10 Medjool dates, pitted
- $^1/_4$ cup shredded, unsweetened coconut
- 1 tablespoon coconut oil
- rind of 1 lemon
- 1 tablespoon freshly-squeezed lemon juice
- $^1/_4$ cup shredded, unsweetened coconut, for rolling

INSTRUCTIONS:

1. Place the cashews in a food processor, and mix until roughly ground so that only tiny pieces remain. Remove from food processor and set aside.

2. In your food processor, mix together the dates, shredded coconut, coconut oil, and lemon rind and mix until the dates are mashed.

3. Add the ground cashews and lemon juice and mix until a ball of dough starts to form.

4. Form into ping-pong sized balls, then roll in shredded coconut.

5. Store in the fridge in an air-tight, glass container for 3–5 days.

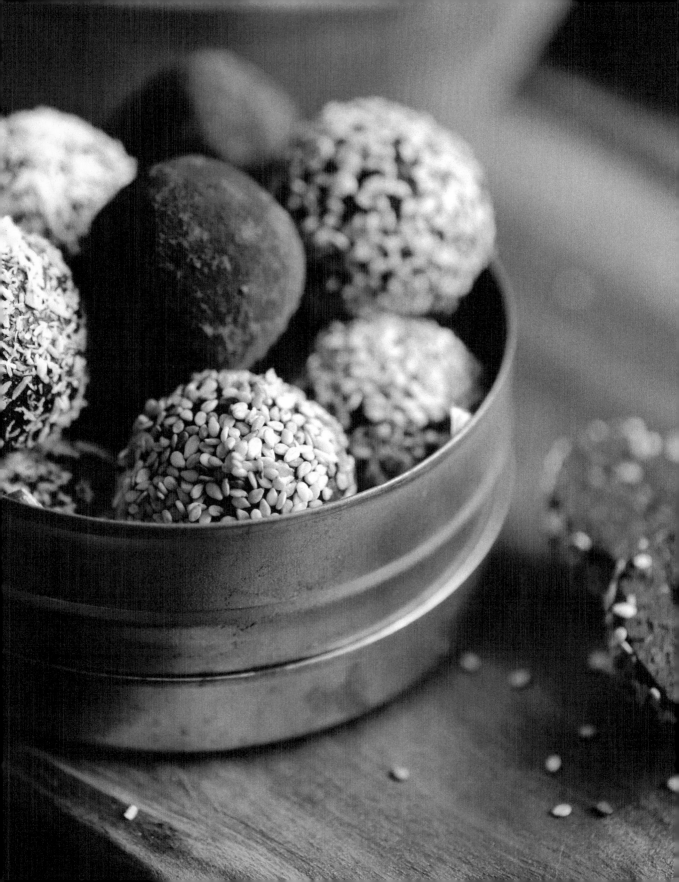

Maca Balls

Makes 18–20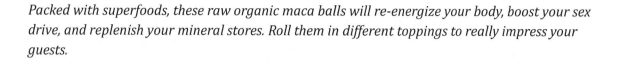

Packed with superfoods, these raw organic maca balls will re-energize your body, boost your sex drive, and replenish your mineral stores. Roll them in different toppings to really impress your guests.

INGREDIENTS:

- $^3/_4$ cup raw cacao powder
- $^1/_4$ cup maca powder
- 1 cup walnuts
- $^1/_2$ cup Medjool dates, soaked
- 2 tablespoons coconut oil, melted
- 1 teaspoon pure vanilla extract
- $^1/_2$ teaspoon sea salt
- 1 $^1/_2$ teaspoons ground cinnamon
- 2 tablespoons real maple syrup
- $^1/_4$ cup each shredded coconut, toasted sesame seeds and raw cacao powder, for rolling

INSTRUCTIONS:

1. Mix all ingredients, except for toppings, in a food processor until a lightly textured dough forms.

2. Shape into ping-pong sized balls, then roll in either coconut, toasted sesame seeds, or cacao powder, or make some of each.

3. Chill in the fridge for at least 30 minutes before serving.

4. Store in the fridge, or better yet the freezer, to stop yourself from eating them all!

Apple Streusel Muffins

Makes 12

These tender, coffee-cake like muffins are the perfect fall snack when served warm and paired with a green tea or a latte. The apple and squash take the place of the butter and sugar normally found in muffins, and provide you with a few extra servings of fruits and vegetables. The crumb topping makes them look super fancy, so they are great for serving to unexpected visitors.

INGREDIENTS:

- $^3/_4$ cup brown rice flour
- $^3/_4$ cup buckwheat flour
- $^1/_2$ cup almond flour
- 1 teaspoon baking soda
- 1 teaspoon baking powder
- 1 teaspoon ground cinnamon
- $^1/_4$ teaspoon ground nutmeg
- $^1/_2$ teaspoon sea salt
- $^1/_4$ cup coconut oil, melted
- 1 large egg
- $^1/_3$ cup unsweetened applesauce
- $^2/_3$ cup real maple syrup
- $^1/_3$ cup water
- $^1/_2$ cup butternut squash puree
- 1 tablespoon apple cider vinegar
- 1 teaspoon pure vanilla extract
- 1 teaspoon freshly grated ginger
- 1 cup grated apple
- $^1/_3$ cup sucanat or coconut sugar
- $^1/_3$ cup gluten-free rolled oats
- 2 small apples, peeled and chopped

INSTRUCTIONS:

1. Preheat oven to 350°F.

2. In a large bowl, whisk together flours, baking soda, baking powder, cinnamon, nutmeg, and sea salt and set aside.

3. In a food processor, mix together coconut oil, egg, applesauce, maple syrup, water, butternut squash, apple cider vinegar, vanilla, and ginger until just combined.

4. Add in flour mixture and blend again briefly until well combined. Add in grated apple and pulse a few times to incorporate.

5. Pour batter into a muffin tin lined with silicone muffin cups, leaving some space at the top for the topping.

6. Sprinkle about $^1/_2$ tablespoon each of sucanat, rolled oats, and chopped apples on top of each muffin.

7. Bake for 30-35 minutes or until tops of muffins are firm to the touch.

> **NOTE:**
>
> Adapted from my mentor Meghan Telpner's Blueberry Muffins. The original recipe can be found here: http://www.meghantelpner.com/blog/blueberry-muffins-and-a-side-of-gratitude/

Carrot Cake

Serves 12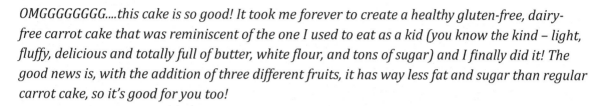

OMGGGGGGGG....this cake is so good! It took me forever to create a healthy gluten-free, dairy-free carrot cake that was reminiscent of the one I used to eat as a kid (you know the kind – light, fluffy, delicious and totally full of butter, white flour, and tons of sugar) and I finally did it! The good news is, with the addition of three different fruits, it has way less fat and sugar than regular carrot cake, so it's good for you too!

INGREDIENTS:

Wet ingredients:
- $^1/_2$ cup applesauce
- $^1/_4$ cup coconut oil
- 3 cups shredded carrots
- 1 cup crushed pineapple
- 4 large eggs
- $^1/_2$ cup coconut sugar
- $^1/_2$ cup raw honey
- 2 teaspoons pure vanilla extract
- 1 teaspoon apple cider vinegar

Dry ingredients:
- $^1/_2$ cup almond flour
- 1 cup brown rice flour
- $^1/_4$ cup quinoa flour
- $^1/_4$ cup arrowroot starch
- 1 teaspoon baking soda
- 1 $^1/_2$ teaspoons ground cinnamon
- 1 $^1/_2$ teaspoons ground nutmeg
- $^1/_2$ teaspoon ground cloves
- $^1/_2$ teaspoon ground ginger

INSTRUCTIONS:

1. Preheat oven to 325°F.
2. In a food processor mix together all wet ingredients until smooth.
3. In a large bowl, whisk together all dry ingredients until well combined.
4. Add the dry ingredients to the wet ingredients and process until combined.
5. Pour batter into a square glass baking pan, and shake slightly to flatten out the top.
6. Bake for 40-50 minutes or until the middle is firm to the touch and cake is cooked through.
7. Remove from oven and let cool.
8. If desired, top with the *Cream Cheese Icing* (from the *Sweet n' Savoury Dips and Dressings* section).

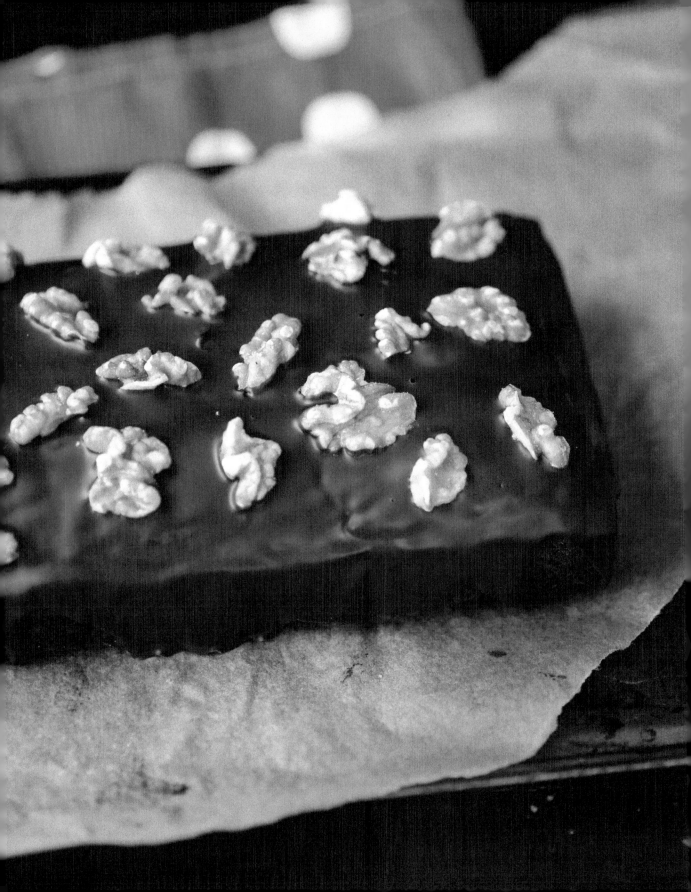

Chocolate-Pumpkin Loaf

Serves 8–10

This loaf is sure to become your new favourite way to eat pumpkin. Low in fat, high in fruit, and absolutely delicious, it is sure to have your kids asking for seconds. Drizzle with the Chocolate-Orange Glaze and serve it as a dessert – or omit the glaze and serve it for breakfast!

INGREDIENTS:

- coconut oil, for greasing the loaf pan
- $1/4$ cup unsweetened applesauce
- 2 tablespoons coconut oil, melted
- $1/3$ cup cocoa powder
- $1/3$ cup plus 2 tablespoons boiling water
- 1 cup pumpkin purée
- 1 cup raw honey
- 1 teaspoon pure vanilla extract
- $1/2$ cup buckwheat flour
- $1/2$ cup brown rice flour
- $1/2$ cup gluten-free oat flour
- $1/2$ teaspoon gound cinnamon
- $1/4$ teaspoon ground nutmeg
- $1/4$ teaspoon ground ground ginger
- $3/4$ teaspoon sea salt
- $2/4$ teaspoon baking soda
- $1/2$ cup dairy-free mini chocolate chips

INSTRUCTIONS:

1. Preheat oven to 350°F. Grease a glass loaf pan with coconut oil.

2. In a food processor, mix together the applesauce, coconut oil, cocoa powder, water, pumpkin purée, honey, and vanilla.

3. In a large mixing bowl, mix together the flours, spices, salt, and baking soda.

4. Add the flour mixture to the pumpkin mixture and mix together until well combined.

5. Stir in the chocolate chips by hand, and pour the batter into the glass loaf pan.

6. Bake for 55–60 minutes, or until the top is firm to touch and loaf is cooked through. Let cool for at least fifteen minutes.

7. If serving as a dessert, spread the *Chocolate-Orange Glaze* (from the *Sweet n' Savoury Dips and Dressings* section) over the top of the loaf, and serve.

8. Store in the fridge in an air-tight container for up to a week.

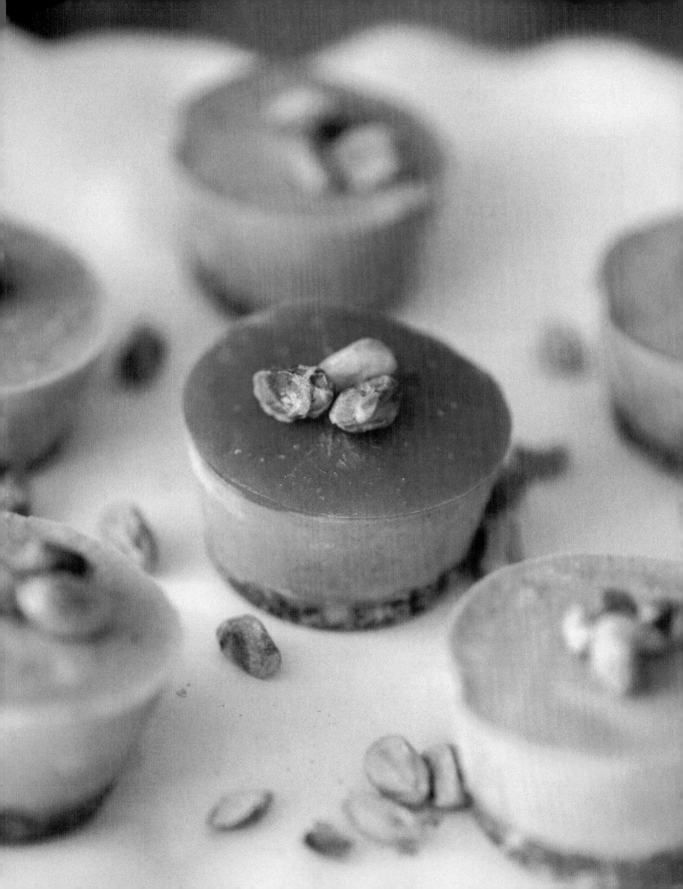

Raw Strawberry Mini Cheesecakes

Makes 6-8 mini cakes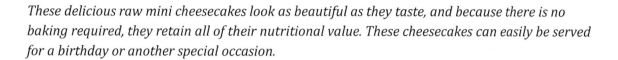

These delicious raw mini cheesecakes look as beautiful as they taste, and because there is no baking required, they retain all of their nutritional value. These cheesecakes can easily be served for a birthday or another special occasion.

INGREDIENTS:

Crust Ingredients:

- $^1/_4$ cup pistachios, roasted and salted
- $^1/_2$ cup cashews (not soaked)
- $^1/_4$ cup Medjool dates, soaked 4–6 hours, then drained
- $^1/_2$ teaspoon extra-virgin olive oil
- $^1/_2$ teaspoon ground cinnamon

Filling Ingredients:

- 1 cup cashews, soaked 4–6 hours, then drained
- $^1/_4$ cup real maple syrup
- 4 Medjool dates
- 2 tablespoons creamed coconut or coconut butter
- 1 tablespoon freshly-squeezed lemon juice
- a pinch of sea salt
- 3 cups frozen strawberries

INSTRUCTIONS:

1. Mix all crust ingredients together in a food processor so that they start to stick together but some texture still remains.

2. On a parchment-paper-lined cookie sheet, press the dough into several round cookie cutters firmly to form mini crusts.

3. Process all filling ingredients together in a food processor until smooth. Pour the filling on top of the crusts. Place the cheesecakes in the freezer to set for at least two hours.

4. Remove the cheesecakes from the freezer and let them sit on the counter for five minutes before serving. If desired, top with homemade strawberry purée.

> **TIP:**
>
> To make fresh strawberry purée, add one cup of frozen strawberries, one tablespoon of maple syrup, and a squeeze of fresh lemon to a large pot and bring to a boil. Reduce heat slightly and continue to cook over medium heat until mixture thickens. Remove from heat, and purée with and immersion blender (or food processor) until smooth. Serve warm or cold.

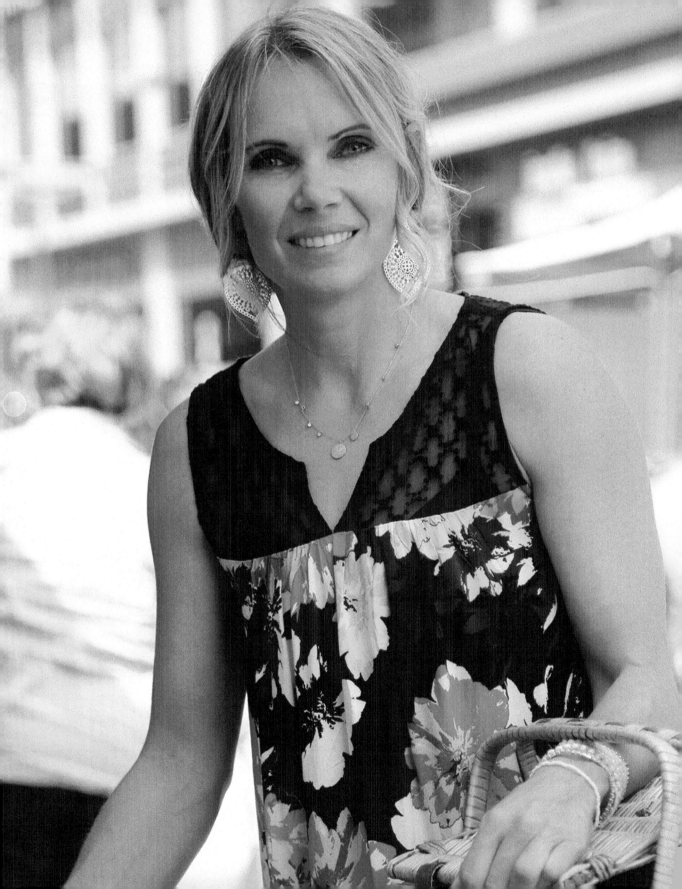

ABOUT THE AUTHOR

Michelle is a Culinary Nutrition Expert, Holistic Health Coach, and Personal Trainer whose passion is teaching people how they can transform their lives through nutrition and exercise. Michelle has written two cookbooks, *Smart Snacking for Sports* and *Help Yourself to Seconds* and is currently working on her third book.

Michelle lives in Ottawa, Canada, with her four children where she loves spending time exploring the outdoors and dreaming up new creations in her kitchen. She shares her knowledge of cooking, nutrition, and fitness on her website www.michellevodrazka.com. For media inquiries or public speaking engagements, please send your request along with relevant details to info@michellevodrazka.com.

Connect with Michelle:

Website: www.michellevodrazka.com

Twitter: https://twitter.com/MomMeFit

Facebook: https://www.facebook.com/michellejulie36

Instagram: https://instagram.com/michellevodrazka/

Linked in: https://www.linkedin.com/in/michelle-vodrazka-11a08a10

REFERENCES

1.   Wansink, Brian. Mindless Eating: Why We Eat More than We Think. New York: Bantam, 2006. Print.

2.   Murray, Sarah. "The World's Biggest Industry." Forbes. Forbes Magazine, 15 Nov. 2007. Web. 18 July 2015. <http://www.forbes.com/2007/11/11/growth-agriculture-business-forbeslife-food07-cx_sm_1113bigfood.html>.

3.   Lustig M.D., Robert. "Still Believe 'A Calorie Is a Calorie'?" The Huffington Post. TheHuffingtonPost.com, 29 Apr. 2013. Web. 18 July 2015. <http://www.huffingtonpost.com/robert-lustig-md/sugar-toxic_b_2759564.html>.

4.   Moss, Michael. Salt, Sugar, Fat: How the Food Giants Hooked Us. New York: Random House, 2013. Print.

5.   Olson, Samantha. "Exercise Reduces Breast Cancer Risk By 50%." Medical Daily. 2 June 2014. Web. 18 July 2015. <http://www.medicaldaily.com/exercise-cuts-breast-cancer-risk-half-better-dieting-285900>.

6.   Office of the Surgeon General (US). "Surgeon General's Call To Action To Prevent and Decrease Overweight and Obesity." Section 1: Overweight and Obesity as Public Health Problems in America. U.S. National Library of Medicine, 2001. Web. 18 July 2015. <http://www.ncbi.nlm.nih.gov/books/NBK44210/>

7.   Greger, Dr. Michael. "The Breast Cancer Survival Vegetable." Breast Cancer Survival Vegetable. 7 Feb. 2014. Web. 18 July 2015. <http://www.care2.com/greenliving/breast-cancer-survival-vegetable.html>

8.   Bianconi, Eva, Allison Piovesan, Federica Facchin, Alina Beraudi, Raffaella Casadei, Flavia Frabetti, Lorenza Vitale, Maria Chiara Pelleri, Simone Tassani, Francesco Piva, Soledad Perez-Amodio, Pierluigi Strippoli, and Silvia Canaider. "An Estimation of the Number of Cells in the Human Body." Annals of Human Biology 40.6 (2013): 463-71. Informa Helthcare.

9.   Pasquella, Cynthia. "You Are What You Eat Is A Big Lie." Cynthia Pasquella Celebrity Nutritionist The Transformational Nutritionist You Are What You Eat Is A Big Lie Comments. Web. 18 July 2015. <http://www.cynthiapasquella.com/you-are-what-you-eat-is-a-big-lie/>.

10.   ibid.

11.   "Sleep Deprivation and Stress: How Stress Affects Sleep." WebMD. WebMD, 10 Mar. 2014. Web. 18 July 2015. <http://www.webmd.com/sleep-disorders/guide/tips-reduce-stress>.

12.   ibid.

13.   Magee, MPH, RD, Elaine. "The Facts About Food Cravings." WebMD. WebMD, 13 Jan. 2005. Web. 18 July 2015. <http://www.webmd.com/diet/the-facts-about-food-cravings>.

14.   Mah CD; Mah KE; Kezirian EJ; Dement WC. The effects of sleep extension on the athletic performance of collegiate basketball players. SLEEP 2011; 34(7):943-950.

15.   Kompf, Justin. "Change Your Clients' Behavior One Habit at a Time." Elite FTS Change Your Clients Behavior One Habit at a Time Comments. 28 Nov. 2012. Web. 18 July 2015. <http://www.elitefts.com/education/training/change-your-clients-behavior-one-habit-at-a-time/>.

16.   "Healthy Fats." Precision Nutrition. 9 Nov. 2009. Web. 7 July 2015. <http://www.precisionnutrition.com/all-about-healthy-fats>.

17.   ibid.

18.   Andrews, Ryan, and Brian St. Pierre. "Forget Calorie Counting: Try This Calorie Control Guide for Men and Women | Precision Nutrition." Precision Nutrition. 25 Sept. 2012. Web. 18 July 2015. <http://www.precisionnutrition.com/calorie-control-guide>.

19.   Jeukendrup, PhD, Asker, and Michael Gleeson, PhD. "Dehydration and Its Effects on Performance." Human-kinetics. Web. 18 July 2015. <http://www.humankinetics.com/excerpts/excerpts/dehydration-and-its-effects-on-performance>.

20.   "TRX Home." TRX Training. Web. 18 July 2015. <https://www.trxtraining.com/products/trx-home>.

21.   Jeukendrup, PhD, Asker, and Michael Gleeson, PhD.

22.   "10,000 Steps - The Walking Site." 10,000 Steps - The Walking Site. Web. 18 July 2015. <http://www.thewalkingsite.com/10000steps.html>.

23.   "21 Quotes From Henry Ford On Business, Leadership And Life." Forbes. Forbes Magazine, 31 Mar. 2013. Web. 7 July 2015. <http://www.forbes.com/sites/erikaandersen/2013/05/31/21-quotes-from-henry-ford-on-business-leadership-and-life/>.

24.   "50 Other Names for Sugar - Organic Authority." Organic Authority. 3 Apr. 2013. Web. 7 July 2015. <http://www.organicauthority.com/health/50-other-names-for-sugar.html>.

25.   "Overweight and Obesity Statistics." Overweight and Obesity Statistics. 1 Oct. 2012. Web. 7 July 2015. <http://www.niddk.nih.gov/health-information/health-statistics/Pages/overweight-obesity-statistics.aspx>.

26.   Oliver, Jamie. "Teach Every Child about Food." 1 Feb. 2010. Web. 18 July 2015. <http://www.ted.com/talks/jamie_oliver.html>.

27.   Thompson, Dennis. "Fat No Longer the Focus of New U.S. Dietary Guidelines." WebMD.

WebMD, 26 June 2015. Web. 8 July 2015. <http://consumer.healthday.com/vitamins-and-nutrition-information-27/dietary-fat-health-news-301/fat-no-longer-focus-of-new-u-s-dietary-guidelines-700798.html>.

28.   Berardi, Ph.D., John. "How to Fix a Broken Diet: 3 Ways to Get Your Eating on Track." Precision Nutrition. 12 June 2013. Web. 8 July 2015. Downey, Sean. "Why Fitness Tracker Calorie Counts Are All Over the Map." Wired.com. Conde Nast Digital, 17 Aug. 2012. Web. 8 July 2015. <http://www.precisionnutrition.com/fix-a-broken-diet>.

29.   "Trans Fat Is Double Trouble for Your Heart Health." Trans Fat: Avoid This Cholesterol Double Whammy. Web. 18 July 2015. <http://www.mayoclinic.org/diseases-conditions/high-blood-cholesterol/in-depth/trans-fat/art-20046114>.

30.   Ferder, Leon, Marcelo Damián Ferder, and Felipe Inserra. "The Role of High-Fructose Corn Syrup in Metabolic Syndrome and Hypertension." Current Hypertension Reports Curr Hypertens Rep (2010): 105-12. Print.

31.   Ruppel Shell, Ellen. "Artificial Sweeteners May Change Our Gut Bacteria in Dangerous Ways." Scientific American Global RSS. 17 Mar. 2015. Web. 18 July 2015. <http://www.scientificamerican.com/article/artificial-sweeteners-may-change-our-gut-bacteria-in-dangerous-ways/>.

32.   Nakanishi, Yuko, Koichi Tsuneyama, Makoto Fujimoto, Thucydides L. Salunga, Kazuhiro Nomoto, Jun-Ling An, Yasuo Takano, Seiichi Iizuka, Mitsunobu Nagata, Wataru Suzuki, Tsutomu Shimada, Masaki Aburada, Masayuki Nakano, Carlo Selmi, and M. Eric Gershwin. "Monosodium Glutamate (MSG): A Villain and Promoter of Liver Inflammation and Dysplasia." Journal of Autoimmunity (2008): 42-50. Print.

33.   "Two Preservatives to Avoid?" 1 Feb. 2011. Web. 18 July 2015. <http://www.berkeleywellness.com/healthy-eating/food-safety/article/two-preservatives-avoid>.

34.   "Food Additives Linked to Health Concerns." EWG. 12 Nov. 2012. Web. 18 July 2015. <http://www.ewg.org/research/ewg-s-dirty-dozen-guide-food-additives/food-additives-linked-health-risks>.

35.   Zengin, N., D. Yüzbaşıoğlu, F. Ünal, S. Yılmaz, and H. Aksoy. "The Evaluation of the Genotoxicity of Two Food Preservatives: Sodium Benzoate and Potassium Benzoate." Food and Chemical Toxicology (2010): 763-69. Print.

36.   "Sulphites - One of the Ten Priority Food Allergens." Health Canada. 26 Oct. 2012. Web. 18 July 2015. <http://www.hc-sc.gc.ca/fn-an/pubs/securit/2012-allergen_sulphites-sulfites/index-eng.php>.

37.   Harrington, Rebecca. "Does Artificial Food Coloring Contribute to ADHD in Children?" Scientific American. 27 Apr. 2015. Web. 18 July 2015. <http://www.scientificamerican.com/article/does-artificial-food-coloring-contribute-to-adhd-in-children/>.

38.   Gold, Mary. "Sustainable Agriculture: Definitions and Terms." Sustainable Agriculture:

Definitions and Terms. 1 Aug. 2007. Web. 18 July 2015. <http://afsic.nal.usda.gov/sustainable-agriculture-definitions-and-terms-1>

39. "Food Additives Linked to Health Concerns." EWG. Web. 18 July 2015. <http://www.ewg.org/research/ewg-s-dirty-dozen-guide-food-additives/food-additives-linked-health-risks>.

40. "EWG." Web. 19 July 2015. <http://www.ewg.org>.

41. "Skin Deep® Cosmetics Database | EWG." Skin Deep Home Comments. Web. 19 July 2015. <http://www.ewg.org/skindeep/>.

42. "EWG's Guide to Healthy Cleaning." Web. 19 July 2015. <http://www.ewg.org/guides/cleaners>.

43. Clark, Melissa. "Olive Oil Granola With Dried Apricots and Pistachios Recipe." NYT Cooking. 10 Jan. 2010. Web. 18 July 2015. <http://cooking.nytimes.com/recipes/1012630-olive-oil-granola-with-dried-apricots-and-pistachios>.

44. Telpner, Meghan. "Yogi Spice Tea." 20 Apr. 2009. Web. 18 July 2015. <http://www.meghantelpner.com/blog/warm-tea-on-a-cold-night/>.

45. Adams, Shelley. Whitewater Cooks: Pure, Simple and Real Creations from the Fresh Tracks Cafe. North Vancouver: Whitecap, 2007. Print.

46. Hill, McKel. "Spinach Basil Pesto." Nutrition Stripped. 5 May 2013. Web. 18 July 2015. <http://nutritionstripped.com/spinach-basil-pesto/>

RECIPE INDEX

200 Foodie Pack: Designed by Freepik and released for Smashing Magazine

CPSIA information can be obtained
at www.ICGtesting.com
Printed in the USA
LVOW01s1406090316

478373LV00030B/196/P